ABORTION PILL REVERSAL

GEORGE DELGADO, MD

Abortion Pill Reversal

A Second Chance at Choice

With a Foreword by Lila Rose

IGNATIUS PRESS   SAN FRANCISCO

Unless otherwise indicated, Scripture quotations are from the Revised Standard Version of the Bible—Second Catholic Edition (Ignatius Edition), copyright © 2006 National Council of the Churches of Christ in the United States of America. Used by permission. All rights reserved worldwide.

Details in some anecdotes and stories have been changed to protect the identity of the persons involved.

This book is not intended to replace the advice and treatment of a medical professional. Readers are encouraged to consult a qualified professional regarding treatment. The author and publisher specifically disclaim liability, loss, or risk, personal or otherwise, that is incurred as a consequence, directly or indirectly, of the use or application of any of the contents of this book.

Cover art and design by Enrique J. Aguilar

© 2025 by Ignatius Press, San Francisco
All rights reserved
ISBN 978-1-62164-810-9 (PB)
ISBN 978-1-64229-364-7 (eBook)
Library of Congress Control Number 2025937952
Printed in the United States of America ∞

I dedicate this book to the many brave women who have attempted abortion pill reversal, especially in the early days, and to my favorite nurse, Liz.

A.M.D.G.

CONTENTS

Foreword by Lila Rose	9
Preface	13
Introduction: Can You Really Reverse an Abortion?	17

Part 1

Chapter 1: How a Family Physician Became a Pioneer	23
Chapter 2: The Key and the False Key: How Mifepristone Abortion Works	33
Chapter 3: The Science of Reversal Made Simple	41
Chapter 4: The Political Agenda That Got Mifepristone Approved	48
Chapter 5: The Growth of the Abortion Pill Industry	54
Chapter 6: Reversal in the United States	68
Chapter 7: It's a Small World	72

Part 2

Chapter 8: "Three Baby Dads—That Doesn't Look Good on You"	85
Chapter 9: God Strengthens	94
Chapter 10: Mimi and Her Baby Girl	98
Chapter 11: A Second Chance	100
Chapter 12: We Are Chosen	104

Chapter 13: From Abortion to Reversal to Public Speaking	114
Chapter 14: Abortion of Twins: "Am I Making the Right Decision or Not?"	118
Chapter 15: From Russia	122
Chapter 16: I Felt Like a Single Parent in a Two-Parent Household	124
Chapter 17: A Grandfather's Perspective	126
Chapter 18: The Very First Known Reversal	128
Chapter 19: Above the Clouds: My Perspective as a Hotline Nurse and Nurse Practitioner	135
Chapter 20: My APR Journey as a Wife and a Nurse	151
Chapter 21: The First APR Hotline Nurse	161
Chapter 22: Dr. Delgado's First APR Case	167
Chapter 23: The First Doctor to Be Banned from Saving Lives	174

Part 3

Chapter 24: Common Themes	193
Chapter 25: What's in a Name?	197
Chapter 26: David Versus Goliath: Why Big Abortion Doesn't Want You to Know About APR	206
Chapter 27: Answering Critics: Would You Ban CPR?	225
Chapter 28: Steno Institute	229
Chapter 29: The Future with APR as the Standard of Care	235
Chapter 30: Final Words	238
Index	243

FOREWORD

Courage is often born in quiet moments. It happens when someone is willing to say yes when the world says no. That's what Dr. George Delgado did. He listened when no one else was listening. He believed when so many had given up hope.

Abortion pill reversal is for women who thought they had no choice—women who took the first abortion pill and then were told that it was too late, that they could not change their minds. But the truth is, they could. And Dr. Delgado was the indispensable man to show them the way.

This book is about what happens when we tell the truth. It is about a simple but powerful reality: Human life begins at the moment of fertilization. Every child in the womb is a human being, created with purpose and dignity, worthy of protection. And every successful abortion ends the life of a human child. That's the hard truth. Every mother has a right to know the full truth about what abortion is and what it does. And every mother deserves to know that there is still hope, even after she takes the first pill in a chemical abortion.

Dr. Delgado never set out to start a movement. He wanted to be a good family doctor, helping patients through pregnancies and illnesses, supporting them through life's challenges. But when a woman called him, desperate and asking for help after taking the first abortion pill, he did not turn her away. He knew about progesterone—how it supports pregnancy, how it could possibly counteract the effects of mifepristone—and so he tried. And it worked. That one yes became thousands of yeses.

The abortion industry does not want people to know this. They want women to believe the lie that abortion is the only option, that once they start, they cannot turn back. They want women to stay silent, to accept regret as the price of so-called choice. But that is not true. Abortion is not empowerment. It is the destruction of a child's life, and it can leave women wounded and alone.

Dr. Delgado's story shines a light into that darkness. He tells the stories of women who were told there was no hope but who found it anyway. He tells the stories of fathers who refused to give up, of nurses and doctors who fought to save babies from the brink of death.

This is the story of Dr. Delgado's quiet courage, of the many people who have joined him, and of the thousands of babies who are alive today because of abortion pill reversal.

This book also shows the brutal reality of the abortion industry—the Medical-Abortion Complex that profits from the destruction of life and fights to keep women in the dark. They don't want women to know about abortion pill reversal because it threatens their bottom line. They are not interested in offering a choice if that choice means choosing life.

Abortion pill reversal gives women a second chance. It is a lifeline for mothers who regret their decisions and want to save their children. And it is a reminder that no situation is hopeless, no decision is final, and no life is disposable.

This book is not just about medical facts or protocols; it is about real people. It is about the women who said, "I want to fight for my baby." It is about the babies who are now growing up in loving homes because someone stood up and said, "Let's try." It is about the fathers and families who stepped in when it mattered most.

Dr. Delgado's story is one of courage, but it is also a story of love. Love for the mother who feels trapped. Love for the child who deserves to live. Love for the truth, even when it is hard to speak.

As you read these pages, I hope you are inspired to speak the truth boldly, to offer hope to the hopeless, and to stand up for life—no matter the cost. Every child matters. Every mother deserves the chance to choose life. And together, we can save every child from abortion and create a future of flourishing families.

Lila Rose
Founder and president, Live Action
June 2025

PREFACE

I felt compelled to write this book in order to speak directly to people about the life-altering, life-saving treatment I named abortion pill reversal. Abortion pill reversal, or APR, gives women who have started the chemical abortion process a second chance at choice. In a nutshell, it is a game changer.

I needed to write this book to help fulfill my mission of increasing awareness, education, and research around APR. Many powerful people and organizations who make up the Medical-Abortion Complex do not want you to know about APR.[1] When women do change their minds after starting their chemical abortions, voices in the Medical-Abortion Complex want them to think that their first decision was irrevocable in an attempt to erase the autonomy of women who want a second chance at choice.

The mainstream media support the Medical-Abortion Complex by limiting information about APR and enabling the echo chamber of misinterpretations of data,

---

[1] See chapter 26 to learn more about the Medical-Abortion Complex. It consists of many interconnected organizations and powerful individuals, with Planned Parenthood at the center. It includes respected medical organizations such as the American College of Obstetricians and Gynecologists (ACOG), the American Medical Association (AMA), and the American Academy of Family Physicians (AAFP). The American Civil Liberties Union (ACLU) and deep-pocketed liberal organizations and individuals defend and protect the complex. US government agencies such as the Food and Drug Administration (FDA), National Institutes of Health (NIH), and United States Agency for International Development (USAID) are biased in favor of and protect abortion.

distortions, and outright lies. This book presents the other side of the matter, sharing the facts, the people, and the stories behind APR, so you can make up your own mind.

I was one of the pioneers of APR; my first reversal was the second documented case. When I helped the woman with my first reversal, I was unaware of Dr. Matthew Harrison's previous case. Later, I started the Abortion Pill Reversal Network, website, and hotline.

I never intended my career path to prepare me to become a researcher or a founder of a movement. I intended only to be the very best family physician I could be. However, God's plans are not man's plans.

The son of Alvaro and Cecilia Delgado, I grew up in Northern California in a family of seven boys of parents who had immigrated from Colombia. I attended medical school at the University of California, Davis, and completed my family medicine residency at UCLA Santa Monica Medical Center. I am board certified in family medicine and hospice and palliative medicine. These specialties have allowed me to care for life at its most vulnerable stages—in the womb and closer to the tomb.

In what turned out to be a preparation for my then-unimagined APR endeavors, I completed the rigorous course in NaProTECHNOLOGY, through which I became an expert in using bioidentical progesterone to treat women with low progesterone levels who were showing signs of impending miscarriage.[2] It was my knowledge of

---

[2] NaProTECHNOLOGY is a new women's health science developed by Dr. Thomas Hilgers and his colleagues. It seeks to treat reproductive system problems such as infertility by diagnosing root causes and treating them, instead of replacing, circumventing, or damaging the reproductive system. Because NaProTECHNOLOGY and the professionals utilizing it respect the integrity of the replicative system and the dignity of patients, it is acceptable to people of all religious and ethical stripes.

progesterone that allowed me to answer yes to the first woman who called asking whether I could help her reverse her chemical abortion.

The story of APR is the story of thousands of courageous women who have decided to exercise their autonomy and make a second choice, a choice for life. APR is also my story and the story of thousands of doctors, mid-level practitioners, nurses, pregnancy help center workers, and ordinary people committed to the ideal that we all deserve second chances.

I hope this book will educate and excite you about what is possible with APR. My goal is for each and every one of you to touch people in your spheres of influence, letting them know that APR is safe and effective and that women given a second chance at choice are very grateful.

INTRODUCTION

Can You Really Reverse an Abortion?

Everyone likes a second chance, because most people have made big decisions in life and later changed their minds. Many have made significant career decisions, damaged personal relationships, behaved recklessly, or purchased large items impulsively, only to later wish they could undo the decisions and reverse course. Sometimes, decisions can be altered; other times, consequences are permanent. Even when consequences are permanent, we often are driven and inspired by hope for a better future, a future enabled by second chances and second choices.

To change our minds is not a sign of weakness; it is a sign of strength. To change our minds, we must be humble enough even to consider that the first decision may have been wrong and wise enough to conclude we made a bad choice. Finally, when the situation demands it, we need the courage to change course.

Whether you consider yourself pro-life, pro-choice, or pro-abortion, I think you will agree that the decision to have an abortion is one of the most difficult, emotionally charged decisions a person can make. Women in these situations often feel helpless and totally forlorn, boxed into a corner with only one obvious exit: abortion. Many feel pressured by others to abort. I have heard countless stories of husbands, boyfriends, ex-boyfriends, and even parents coercing women to abort or threatening to abandon them if they do not.

Once a surgical abortion starts, there is no turning back. However, with chemical abortions, there is a window of opportunity when a woman can change her mind and not only stop but actually reverse the chemical abortion. That is correct: We can reverse the chemical abortion process, snatching the life of the preborn baby from the jaws of death. In saving that life and honoring the wish of the mother seeking the reversal, we give her a new lease on life, emotionally, psychologically, and spiritually.

From the start, it is important to emphasize that those, like me, who offer to help women seek a second chance at choice only propose this life-saving treatment—never impose it. We respect the dignity and sanctity of every human life, preborn or already born, as well as the free will that accompanies that life. We offer education, insight, and guidance, never seeking to coerce.

While we in the abortion pill reversal movement love and honor both the mother and the preborn baby, such is not always the case with those who offer abortions. Stories of misinformation and lies told to women at abortion centers are commonplace. Countless times, we have been told that pregnant women have not been allowed to see their babies on ultrasound. Several years ago, an APR patient shared her story by text: "At the Planned Parenthood clinic I was treated very coldly to say the least, like a cow in a chute waiting to be branded. The dirty deed waiting to be committed and then on to the next, like it was no big deal. Insensitive to the fact that I was about ready to make the worst, most life-altering decision I would forever regret and haunt me for the rest of my days."

This book is about offering women a second chance at choice. In part 1, you will learn what chemical abortion (also called medical abortion, pill abortion, or medication abortion) is and how APR reverses that type of abortion. I will take you through the fascinating story of the birth and development of APR. Additionally, you will get a peek at the corrupt political process that allowed chemical abortion to be approved in the United States. You will see how abortion is big business and how the abortion industry has grown. I will also review the state of APR in the United States and around the world—more than 93 countries and counting.

In part 2, you will read the firsthand accounts of amazing women who have been through the APR process. They first initiated an abortion but then chose reversal. You will learn about the challenges they faced as they changed their minds and started the abortion pill reversal process.

You will also read the account of a father whose preborn baby was saved by APR. You will learn how he grew into manhood and was transformed into the protector he was meant to be. A grandfather also shares his unique perspective.

In addition, Dr. Matthew Harrison will tell his story of the very first abortion pill reversal, the start of a revolution. Three former APR hotline nurses will give you rare glimpses of the challenges, frustrations, triumphs, and joys of APR from their unique perspectives. Terri Palmquist, the pro-life advocate who got me started in APR when she asked me whether I could help a woman who was seeking to reverse her chemical abortion, gives her account of that early case, my first ever. Finally, you will read Dr. Dermot Kearney's story, "The First Doctor to Be Banned from Saving Lives".

Many challenges confronted those who shared their stories, whether they were pioneers or more recent heroes. The many brave doctors, nurses, and advocates who devised a totally novel treatment, because they were deeply committed to help the women who were desperately seeking to undo their chemical abortions, likewise met great obstacles.

These selfless people made a huge, enduring difference in the lives of others.

In part 3, I will summarize some common themes I and others have perceived in APR stories and present the meanings of some of the names that have been given to APR babies. Additionally, I will address why Big Abortion does not want you to know about APR, explain how APR and CPR are quite similar, and provide a glimpse into the future with APR as the standard of care for women who change their minds about their chemical abortions.

The concluding chapter is from the heart, as I explore how APR is truly a metaphor for forgiveness, transformation, and second chances. Women seeking reversal are sometimes criticized, ostracized, and threatened by those who wanted them to abort in the first place. In the early days of APR, these women had to trust that the treatment they would undergo would be safe for them and their preborn babies. They put their faith in their doctors, nurse practitioners, physician assistants, midwives, nurses, and counselors. Ultimately, they trusted themselves and God.

Part 1

I

How a Family Physician Became a Pioneer

It was in the late 1990s when I first heard of a drug called RU-486, which was being studied to be used as an abortion pill—a pill that would replace surgical abortions. It had already been approved in Europe and was gaining traction there. I learned that it blocks the actions of progesterone, the female hormone that is essential for the maintenance of a pregnancy. It was approved in the United States in the year 2000 and was known as mifepristone, with the brand name Mifeprex. In Europe, the brand name is Mifegyne; in Canada, it is called Mifegymiso.

The Phone Call

In 2008, I was seeing patients in my family medicine office in San Diego, California, when I received a phone call from Terri Palmquist that would forever change my life. Terri, a sidewalk counselor in Bakersfield, California, had a website and a toll-free number that people from all over the country could call (see chapter 22 for Terri's story). That day, a woman in Texas reached out to Terri with a unique request. The woman had started the chemical abortion process by taking mifepristone but had changed her mind. She wanted to know whether Terri could help her stop the abortion in order to save her preborn baby.

Terri had never heard of such a thing. As she had done a few other times when she had medical questions, Terri called me. I told Terri that I likewise had never heard of anyone reversing the effects of mifepristone and stopping a chemical abortion. However, I told her I would think about whether it could be done. In my brain were two related but distinct data banks that needed to be bridged: my knowledge of how mifepristone works by blocking the effects of progesterone and my experience using progesterone to prevent miscarriage.

In 2003, two years before my family and I moved from the Bay Area to San Diego County, I had completed the medical consultant program offered by Dr. Thomas Hilgers and his team at the Saint Paul VI Institute. Dr. Hilgers had been using progesterone for years to treat infertility, postpartum depression, and threatened miscarriage.

Threatened miscarriage is when a pregnant woman is having cramping or bleeding—signs that she may lose the baby. I had treated many pregnant women with low progesterone levels who were cramping and/or bleeding by giving them progesterone supplements. In many of those cases, I was able to prevent miscarriages, always using bioidentical progesterone—progesterone that is molecularly identical to that produced by the human body.

On that day, as I pondered Terri's request, God made the connection in my mind. The pregnant woman in Texas who had taken mifepristone was in a situation analogous to that of a pregnant woman with low progesterone who is at risk for miscarriage. In both situations, progesterone effects were low—in one case because progesterone was being blocked and in the other because progesterone levels were deficient. I quickly reasoned that I could give the woman who wanted a second chance at choice supplemental progesterone to make up for the progesterone that was being blocked. I knew that in many biological systems, molecules compete for receptors. The one with the higher concentration of molecules often wins. I knew what we needed to do, but now I had to figure out how to do it.

In those days, I was mostly using injectable progesterone, following the protocols that Dr. Hilgers had developed over many years. The reversal of mifepristone, however, would probably require higher or more frequent doses, at least for the first few days while the mifepristone was still in the body battling with the progesterone. Based on this deduction, I devised a protocol using Dr. Hilgers' doses but given more frequently. I would recommend 200 mg progesterone injected once a day for three days, every other day for six doses, and then twice a week until the end of the first trimester, when the placenta is usually producing enough progesterone to sustain the pregnancy.

The next hurdle was geography. The woman was more than seven hundred miles from San Diego. I checked on the internet to see if I could find a doctor in Texas who had been trained in NaProTECHNOLOGY. Fortunately, when I called Dr. Jonnalyn Belocura, she was in the office, had progesterone, and was willing to help. Dr. Belocura agreed to see the patient and use the protocol that I recommended. Terri then reached out to the patient and told her to go to Dr. Belocura's office as soon as possible.

Over the next weeks, I eagerly awaited progress reports that Dr. Belocura, with her patient's permission, would send me. The baby was still alive, and things looked promising. I was overjoyed when I received the news that the mother had delivered a healthy baby girl at term. About a year and a half later, Terri was able to meet that special mother, and she took a picture with her and her precious toddler. They sent that picture to me with an inscription: "Thank you, Dr. Delgado."

After that case, I really did not think much more would come of it. I had helped a person in need, a woman who desperately wanted to stop her chemical abortion, and it worked. Over time, however, I started to receive phone calls from clinics and doctors across the country wanting advice on how to help other women who wanted a second chance at choice. I considered gathering information on these cases and publishing an article in the medical literature so that other medical practitioners might know that reversing mifepristone abortions was often possible.

In 2011, we learned of a woman in the San Francisco Bay Area who wanted to stop her chemical abortion. I called my colleague, Dr. Mary Davenport, who practiced in the East Bay. She agreed to help the woman. Unfortunately, we were not successful in saving the woman's baby. Afterward, Dr. Davenport suggested that I write a case series report for the medical literature. I told her that I had been thinking about doing just that and knew that now was the time to stop procrastinating.

As my coauthor, Dr. Davenport helped me write the first paper in the medical literature on abortion pill reversal. Previously, I had done a great deal of writing for general audiences, including magazines and a weekly newspaper column called Family Health Matters, in the *Benicia Herald*, a small paper in the Bay Area. Medical articles, however, were a whole different animal in terms of the research required.

While I was researching cases for the article, Dr. Davenport shared with me that there had actually been a reversal case before mine. In 2006 in North Carolina, Dr. Matthew Harrison carried out the first known reversal of mifepristone. He reasoned, just as I had, that giving his patient supplemental progesterone might negate the effects of mifepristone. It worked: A beautiful, healthy girl was born after the successful reversal. (Dr. Harrison and I eventually became collaborators, great friends, and confidants; he is a true hero, and his story is in chapter 18.)

Dr. Davenport and I published our paper in 2012 in a peer-reviewed medical journal.[1] In that 2012 paper, we reported on six attempted reversal cases. Four of them were successful, and there were no birth defects, complications, or serious side effects. We thought we were on to something that would be a game changer for women and anticipated that with the article published, more and more pregnant women who had taken mifepristone would learn about the possibility of reversal and might want to attempt it. That being said, I knew we had two problems: (1) women in these situations needed to learn about the possibility of reversal quickly, because time is of the essence, and (2) we needed to have medical practitioners who were available, capable, and willing to help, not just in San Diego but all over the country.

A Network of Providers

With those two challenges in mind, in 2012 I formally launched a network called Abortion Pill Reversal, with the financial support and approval of Culture of Life Family Services (COLFS), the not-for-profit, pro-life organization where I have my medical practice. Vita La Fond, one of the COLFS volunteers, helped with phone calls from clients as our first hotline operator. Soon thereafter,

---

[1] George Delgado and Mary L. Davenport, "Progesterone Use to Reverse the Effects of Mifepristone", *Annals of Pharmacotherapy* 46, no. 12 (2012), https://doi.org/10.1345/aph.1R252.

an intrepid registered nurse, Debbie Bradel, became the hotline nurse and later the first director. We learned as we developed, and we further developed what we learned.

I wanted a name that was descriptive, self-explanatory, medically accurate, and catchy enough to appeal to women in these tough situations. I knew that Planned Parenthood, on its website, had referred to mifepristone abortions as "pill abortions". Abortion pill reversal, abbreviated APR, stuck.

Some questioned the term, arguing that the chemical abortions are prevented, not reversed. However, there is now solid scientific evidence that the abortion process does indeed begin with the ingestion of mifepristone but is stopped and reversed with progesterone (see chapter 3).

We built a website so women would have an easily accessible resource for factual, unbiased information before, during, or after a chemical abortion. Good information is crucial to the informed consent process, something that was a high priority for us. We wanted to be sure that we educated and proposed but never imposed our moral convictions on others. The information we provided on chemical abortion itself was more complete and more accurate than what we found on the websites of abortion providers.

Connected to the site was a toll-free hotline number that a woman in need could call twenty-four hours a day, seven days a week. Until we recruited more nurses, Debbie Bradel, RN, handled all the phone calls. She has helped hundreds of women with a sweet, loving, authentic, nonjudgmental approach. My wife, Liz Delgado, RN, was the second hotline nurse, and by the time she retired from the hotline in 2023, she had been the longest-serving hotline nurse.

The toll-free hotline number has a collaborative story associated with it. Roger Lopez, a San Diego pro-life hero, was in charge of a group affiliated with Helpers of God's

Precious Infants. Roger and his group would pray in front of abortion centers. He and other trained counselors would also ask women and couples entering the abortion centers whether they needed help. Additionally, Roger had a Grasshopper toll-free number so that he and his team could be available to anyone who needed assistance at any time. Once he knew we needed a toll-free number, he donated it to us. Roger's old number was passed on to Heartbeat International, and it remains the main hotline number today.

One half of the equation was providing ready access to women seeking reversal. The other half was having the medical practitioners ready to assist them. In the early years, every case resulted in a mad scramble as we called pregnancy help centers, doctors I knew, or Church diocesan offices in hopes of finding medical practitioners to treat these women. Precious treatment time was lost as we made call after call, searching for that qualified, compassionate clinician who could treat the woman seeking to reverse her abortion.

We realized we needed to educate and recruit medical practitioners. Initially, we targeted obstetrician gynecologists and family physicians. It was clear early on that pro-life doctors were the most interested and the ones most willing to help. Following Sutton's Law (Willie Sutton said he robbed banks because that's where the money is), I began recruiting doctors from pro-life organizations. Additionally, I started giving talks at conferences and meetings, wherever they would have me. We also had booths at conferences held by the Catholic Medical Association (CMA), Heartbeat International, and other groups.

At the time, Dr. Davenport was a member of the board of directors of the American Association of Pro-Life Obstetricians and Gynecologists (AAPLOG). The other board members were excited about our work and invited me to become the first family physician to sit on their board.

Since then, I have presented at several AAPLOG meetings, giving updates on the progress we have made in abortion pill reversal. AAPLOG and its leaders have been very supportive over the years, and I am quite indebted to them.

Culture of Life Family Services; its board; its forward-thinking chairman, Bill Goyette; and then-CEO Scott Maxwell were instrumental in helping APR grow in the ensuing years. Their guidance, advice, and financial support allowed the organic development of APR to continue.

An enthusiastic team of employees, including Debbie Bradel and Sarah Littlefield, helped grow APR in the early years. Volunteers played a big role in recruiting and vetting physicians for the network, almost acting like a credentialing service. The late Gene Villinski was especially enthusiastic, energetic, and effective in that regard. Gene created a computer map of the United States with virtual pins marking where we had APR Network doctors.

In 2018, my colleagues and I authored a large case series study that was published in a peer-reviewed medical journal.[2] We analyzed the data of 547 patients who had attempted reversal of their chemical abortions (see chapter 3 for more on that paper). That study brought definite credibility to APR because of the large numbers of subjects and the effectiveness of the high-dose progesterone protocol at reversing chemical abortions.[3] Probably because it was so impactful, it was met by a great deal of resistance and criticism by supporters of abortion (see chapter 26 on opposition to APR).

---

[2] George Delgado, Steven J. Condly, Mary Davenport, Thidarat Tinnakornsrisuphap, Jonathan Mack, Veronica Khauv et al., "A Case Series Detailing the Successful Reversal of the Effects of Mifepristone Using Progesterone", *Issues in Law & Medicine* 33, no. 1 (2018): 3–14.

[3] Initially, I recommended using injected progesterone. After our 2018 study, I switched to what I termed the "high-dose oral" protocol (see chapter 3 on why that change occurred).

One of the big issues involved the prestudy review by the institutional review board (IRB). The role of the IRB is to protect subjects in studies from any harm. One of our coauthors, Jonathan Mack, PhD, RN-BC, is a faculty member in the Hahn School of Nursing and Health Science at the University of San Diego (USD). Because of his involvement in the study, we were able to use USD's IRB, and it approved the study by granting an exemption to a detailed review because the risk of harm to the subjects was minimal.

Once the study was published, USD received a fair amount of negative publicity, a glaring light it did not expect or want. People there looked at the application and the study and pointed out that we had inadvertently included data outside the time frame the IRB had approved. Because of that minor technicality, USD revoked the IRB approval. Therefore, we had to withdraw the paper from the journal.

We moved quickly to submit a new IRB application, this time to a group called Aspire, because USD refused to accept a corrected application. Aspire approved the study, and we were able to republish the article. Even though the study was essentially approved by two IRBs, the other side persisted in spreading the lie that we had "an ethics problem".

Over time, the financial strain of what had become a national organization was more than the local nonprofit could bear. Culture of Life Family Services transferred the network to Heartbeat International in April 2018. Heartbeat rebranded the program as Abortion Pill Rescue. I still use the term *abortion pill reversal* for the process of reversing the effects of mifepristone to stop a medical abortion.

As of June 2025, there are more than 1,400 doctors, other medical practitioners, and clinics in the Abortion Pill Rescue Network (APRN). We have helped women in all 50 states and in at least 93 other countries. Additionally, there are now regional networks in Australia, Switzerland, Russia, and the United Kingdom. These regional networks are beneficial for overcoming time zone and language barriers. Also, regional organizers have more local contacts and connections, which enables them to recruit medical practitioners for their networks.

Now my involvement in abortion pill reversal is twofold: I serve as a medical adviser to the APRN and continue to oversee research and protocol refinement. To further those goals, I established the Steno Institute in 2018 (see chapter 28 for more information).

APR started with two doctors helping two women who came to them with cries for help. It has grown organically because of the efforts and commitments of thousands of people who believe that life is inherently good and that people should have second choices.

2

The Key and the False Key: How Mifepristone Abortion Works

Researchers have been searching for reliable ways to use drugs to cause abortions for many years. Some described this as pursuing "the holy grail". This chapter will review the history of the development of mifepristone as a method for chemical abortion.

Mifepristone, previously called RU-486, causes abortions by blocking the effects of progesterone, the female hormone that is vital for pregnancy. The word *progesterone* says what this chemical does: *Pro* means "for"; *gest* means "gestation" (pregnancy). The hormone progesterone maintains the pregnancy by developing and maintaining the uterine lining so that it is receptive to the five-to-seven-day-old human embryo traveling down the fallopian tube seeking to find a stable home for nine months. Normal progesterone levels and function are important, even before the baby is conceived.

After conception, this essential hormone causes the placenta to adhere firmly to the lining of the uterus. I call it the superglue of the placenta. A very close connection between the placenta and the lining of the uterus is essential for the embryo, and later fetus, to receive oxygen, water, and nutrients from the mother. Likewise, a tight seal is imperative for the transfer of carbon dioxide and waste products from the baby to the mother.

Besides ensuring that the placenta thrives, progesterone inhibits the production of prostaglandins, potent natural chemicals that cause the uterus to contract. During pregnancy, the uterus, which is essentially a sac made of muscle, must be soft and pliable in order to stretch to accommodate its growing passenger. Contractions, the powerful squeezing of the uterine muscle, are useful only at the time of delivery. They are harmful and can lead to miscarriage or preterm delivery if they occur before the fetus is full term. Prostaglandins and similar chemicals called prostaglandin analogs are used to induce labor.

Progesterone, aside from preventing prostaglandin production, keeps the muscular layer of the uterus in a relaxed state. Additionally, it keeps the opening of the uterus, the cervix, closed so that the inside world does not have contact with the outside world, except through the mother and the placenta. The cervix is essentially a biologic valve, a gate that needs to be kept closed to maintain a pregnancy.

By blocking progesterone, mifepristone has several effects, most notably the separation of the placenta from the lining of the uterus; the superglue is dissolved. With that, the lifeline is cut—fluid and nutrition can no longer reach the preborn baby. This is the primary cause of the death of a preborn baby during a mifepristone chemical abortion. Other effects of mifepristone include the opening of the cervix and the beginning of uterine contractions.

True Keys and False Keys

Dr. Étienne-Émile Baulieu, called "the father of the abortion pill" by *The New York Times* and others, discovered the progesterone receptor in 1970 at the University of Paris.[1] Regarding his work to find a way to produce a chemical abortion, he stated, "The receptors are like a keyhole, and we were trying to produce a false key."[2]

Indeed, keys and keyholes make an excellent analogy for hormone physiology. Imagine that progesterone is a key and that the progesterone receptor (the place where the progesterone molecule lands) is a lock. The key enters the lock and turns it; then the door opens. The door opening represents the hormone effect: the good and necessary physiologic action accomplished by the hormone messenger.

Think of a time when you inserted a key into a lock but the lock would not turn. The key that fits into the lock but will not unlock the door can be considered a false key. That's exactly what mifepristone is—a false key. It enters the lock but blocks the hormone effect by not allowing the door to open.

Fortunately, in the body false keys do not remain in the locks permanently. There is a dynamic state of keys moving in and out of locks. In an effort to reverse a chemical abortion, supplemental progesterone is administered, flooding locks with the true keys, the "good guys", in order to outcompete the false keys, the "bad guys".

How Is a Mifepristone Abortion Performed?

Mifepristone abortion is actually a two-drug process involving the main drug, mifepristone, and a second drug,

---

[1] Pam Belluc, "The Father of the Abortion Pill", *New York Times*, January 17, 2023.

[2] Étienne-Émile Baulieu, quoted in Steven Greenhouse, "A New Pill, a Fierce Battle", *New York Times Magazine*, February 12, 1989, https://www.nytimes.com/1989/02/12/magazine/a-new-pill-a-fierce-battle.html.

taken between twenty-four and forty-eight hours later, called misoprostol (its brand name is Cytotec). The progesterone we give to reverse medical abortion acts only against the mifepristone; it is not an antidote for the misoprostol. All our studies to date have been in women who have taken the mifepristone only, not the misoprostol.

In the United States, mifepristone is given in an oral dose of 200 mg, at up to ten weeks of pregnancy. This dose was previously required to be given in a supervised setting, generally in the presence of a medical practitioner who was certified to dispense mifepristone. However, in 2021, during the COVID-19 pandemic, the Biden administration loosened the restrictions for mifepristone, allowing it to be ordered via telehealth encounters and dispensed by mail-order pharmacies. The requirement for an in-person visit was abolished for the first time, putting the health and lives of women at risk (see chapters 4 and 5).

In the case of both telehealth and in-office treatments for mifepristone abortions, the woman is given one 200 mg mifepristone pill and four 200 mcg misoprostol pills. She is instructed to take the four pills by placing them under the tongue or between the cheek and gums between twenty-four and forty-eight hours after the ingestion of the first pill, the mifepristone. The misoprostol is taken that way to decrease diarrhea and nausea.

The abortion occurs at home, usually in the bathroom. Supporters of medical abortion say that having an abortion in the privacy of one's own home is a great advance. Others feel that having the abortion in a bathroom without any medical help is a disservice to the woman. The reality is that a woman is often alone and forlorn when faced with the prospect of flushing her preborn baby's remains down the toilet. The pain, bleeding, and risks of complications are all borne at home, without medical assistance available. There is no dignity there, for the baby or the mother.

The Abortion Pill Is Different from the Morning-After Pill

Before we dive more deeply, I want to clear up a very common misconception. I have been surprised over the years that even many doctors do not know the difference between the abortion pill (mifepristone) and the morning-after pill, also called emergency contraception and Plan B. The morning-after pill is, in most cases, a high dose of a hormonal contraceptive that a woman takes within seventy-two hours of so-called unprotected intercourse in order to prevent a pregnancy. There is emerging evidence that the morning-after pill is actually frequently abortifacient because it can change the lining of the uterus to prevent the five-to-seven-day-old embryo from implanting. Although the morning-after pill may cause very early abortions, the intent of the woman taking it is to prevent pregnancy.

The abortion pill, on the other hand, is taken by a woman who knows she is pregnant with the intention of ending her pregnancy. Mifepristone is approved to be taken as late as ten weeks in the pregnancy in order to cause an abortion. It is taken instead of having a surgical abortion.

Statistics in the United States and Around the World

Abortion statistics can be difficult to compile in the United States. States and other jurisdictions are not required to report abortion numbers to the US Centers for Disease

Control and Prevention (CDC). In fact, three jurisdictions that have among the highest abortion numbers—California, Maryland, and New Jersey—do not provide statistics to the CDC. The Guttmacher Institute, the research arm of Planned Parenthood, provides the most reliable abortion statistics for the country. Guttmacher estimated that in 2023, 63 percent of all US abortions were chemical abortions, with the vast majority employing mifepristone.[3] Since there are about one million abortions annually in the United States, that means that more than six hundred thousand are caused by mifepristone.

In some European countries, such as Finland, Norway, and Sweden, mifepristone abortions account for 90 percent of all abortions, according to Guttmacher.[4] The trend worldwide, as in the United States, is an increase in the percentage of chemical abortions.

History of Mifepristone

Dr. Baulieu served as a consultant to French pharmaceutical giant Roussel Uclaf (RU) and helped develop mifepristone. Ten short years later, Dr. George Teutsch, the Roussel Uclaf chief chemist, synthesized the chemical that would later be known as mifepristone. The company gave it the developmental label of RU 486 because it was the 38,486th

---

[3] "Monthly Abortion Provision Study", US Abortion Provision Dashboard, Guttmacher Institute, accessed April 3, 2025, https://www.guttmacher.org/monthly-abortion-provision-study.

[4] Gilda Sedgh and Irum Taqi, "Mifepristone for Abortion in a Global Context: Safe, Effective and Approved in Nearly 100 Countries", Policy Analysis, July 2023, Guttmacher Institute, https://www.guttmacher.org/2023/07/mifepristone-abortion-global-context-safe-effective-and-approved-nearly-100-countries.

chemical in its library of potential drugs. Since the drug was so notorious, the name RU-486 became well known.[5]

Mifepristone was marketed in France after its approval by the French government in 1988. However, due to pro-life pressures and threats of boycotts, Roussel Uclaf CEO Dr. Edouard Sakiz stopped the sale of mifepristone, fearing that his giant company would suffer because of it. At the same time, Hoechst AG, the German pharmaceutical corporation and majority owner of Roussel Uclaf, did not favor marketing an abortion pill. The French government stepped in and forced the company to sell mifepristone in France.[6]

Seeking to avoid corporate liability and protests, Roussel Uclaf transferred the US rights to mifepristone to the Population Council, a pro-abortion advocacy group. In turn, it granted the rights to Danco Laboratories, which was created to be a single-drug pharmaceutical company. A similar strategy was devised for Europe, with Roussel Uclaf granting the rights to Exelgyn, another single-drug pharmaceutical company. The logic was clear: A catastrophic lawsuit would take out only one drug instead of an entire pharmaceutical portfolio. The risky drug was well insulated. The drug was approved in the United States in 2000.[7] (See chapter 4 to find out how mifepristone was approved in the United States.)

The past corporate history of Hoechst AG is interesting, if not eerie. Hoechst AG and its corporate ancestors can be traced back to the 1800s in Germany.[8] In 1916, Hoechst AG was one of the founders and corporate constituents of IG Farben, whose managers were tried at Nuremberg for

---

[5] Greenhouse, "A New Pill, a Fierce Battle".
[6] Ibid.
[7] Ibid.
[8] Amy Tikkanen, ed., "Hoechst Aktiengesellschaft", *Brittanica Money*, accessed June 4, 2025, https://www.britannica.com/money/Hoechst-Aktiengesellschaft.

exploitation of and experimentation on prisoners in Nazi Germany. Furthermore, an IG Farben subsidiary distributed Zyklon B, the cyanide gas used to kill more than one million concentration camp prisoners before and during World War II.[9]

Compared to surgical abortions, methods of which include suction, D&C, D&E, and intact extraction, mifepristone and chemical abortions using other drugs lead to the same results: ending the pregnancy and the life of the preborn baby. In every type of abortion, the mother is also a victim; her fear is exploited by those in the Medical-Abortion Complex, who profit from her abortion. The difference between surgical abortion and mifepristone abortion is that with mifepristone abortion, a woman who changes her mind during the abortion process has a window of opportunity to change course.

---

[9] Amy Tikkanen, ed., "IG Farben", *Brittanica*, accessed June 4, 2025, https://www.britannica.com/topic/IG-Farben; Laura Lati, "IG Farben: Giant of the German Chemical Industry and Participant in Nazi Atrocities", accessed June 4, 2025, https://learncheme.com/wp-content/uploads/Prausnitz/HistoryofChemicalCompaniesProducts/IGFarben.pdf.

3

The Science of Reversal Made Simple

Thus far, colleagues and I have published three articles—and one is awaiting publication—concerning abortion pill reversal in the peer-reviewed medical literature. Other groups have published at least three other studies. *Peer-reviewed* means that other physicians or scientists in related fields have reviewed the research articles and approved them as worthy of publication. The first published article was a small case series documenting the successful reversal of four of six medical abortions.[1] This was what really got the ball rolling and excited people. After that, my colleagues and I started collecting information (with clients' permission) on mifepristone reversals that were reported to the network.

Once we had enough data, we received clearance from an institutional review board (IRB) to publish a much larger case series. This article, published in another peer-review journal, looked at 547 patients who had attempted reversal of mifepristone abortions.[2] It documented that our

---

[1] George Delgado and Mary L. Davenport, "Progesterone Use to Reverse the Effects of Mifepristone", *Annals of Pharmacotherapy* 46, no. 12 (2012), https://doi.org/10.1345/aph.1R252. (The article is available at stenoinstitute.org/resources.)

[2] George Delgado, Steven J. Condly, Mary Davenport, Thidarat Tinnakornsrisuphap, Jonathan Mack, Veronica Khauv et al., "A Case Series Detailing the Successful Reversal of the Effects of Mifepristone Using Progesterone", *Issues in Law & Medicine* 33, no. 1 (2018): 3–14. (The article is available at stenoinstitute.org/resources.)

best protocols were successful and led to births 64–68 percent of the time. This compares to an expected embryo survival rate of 25 percent if mifepristone alone is taken and no treatment is offered. For all the women in the study, the reversal rate was 48 percent. This was significantly lower than our best protocols because some women stopped the progesterone early, took only a few doses, or were given lower doses. Still, 48 percent is statistically and clinically significantly better than the 25 percent expected survival rate if no treatment is offered.

We were especially relieved to see that the birth defect rate was no greater than the birth defect rate in the general population. In the United States, the major birth defect rate is approximately 4 percent.[3] A major birth defect is a defect, present at birth, that requires treatment or that hinders function. That means that out of 100 births, on average, there will be 4 babies with major birth defects. In our 2018 study, the birth defect rate was 2.7 percent.[4]

We found that our preterm delivery rate was lower than the general population. A preterm birth is a delivery prior to 37 weeks of pregnancy. The US preterm birth rate is estimated to be 10 percent.[5] Our rate was 2.7 percent.[6] It is possible that some preterm births occur because of low progesterone. Therefore, an added bonus, besides reversing the abortions, was preventing preterm births in some pregnancies.

---

[3] Erin B. Stallings, Jennifer L. Isenburg, Rachel E. Rutkowski, Russell S. Kirby, Wendy N. Nembhard, Theresa Sandidge et al., "National Population-Based Estimates for Major Birth Defects, 2016–2020", *Birth Defects Research* 116, no. 1 (2024): e2301, https://doi.org/10.1002/bdr2.2301.

[4] Delgado et al., "A Case Series", 3–14.

[5] "Preterm Birth," Maternal Health, US Centers for Disease Control and Prevention, accessed April 5, 2025, https://www.cdc.gov/maternal-infant-health/preterm-birth/.

[6] Delgado et al., "A Case Series", 3–14.

Earlier, I listed an embryo survival rate of up to 25 percent if a pregnant mother takes mifepristone only and does not receive reversal therapy. How do I know that? In 2017, Dr. Mary Davenport did some interesting research that she published in a peer-reviewed journal.[7] She looked at the early mifepristone research, before misoprostol was added to the abortion protocol. Some of those early studies used ultrasound to determine whether the embryo had died. If the embryo was still alive, a surgical abortion would be performed.

In those studies, the embryo survival rate might have been overestimated because some of them waited as little as one day before performing surgical abortions on the embryos that still had heartbeats. Nonetheless, the information is as good as we will get. The embryo survival range after exposure to mifepristone alone was 10–23 percent.

In our subsequent research, we have decided to err on the high side of predicted embryo survival if no treatment is offered, in order to preempt criticism of our analysis of data. That is why we use 25 percent as a historic control.

It was research for our 2018 study that led us to transition from injected progesterone to oral progesterone. In private discussions with Dr. Thomas Hilgers, one of the world's leading experts on the use of progesterone in pregnancy, he shared his belief that progesterone was most effective if delivered by intramuscular injection. However, the injections have a major limitation; they can be uncomfortable—a literal pain in the behind. The off-the-shelf progesterone for injection comes in a 50 mg/ml concentration. Therefore, a standard dose of 200 mg requires a total of 4 ml to

---

[7] Mary Davenport, George Delgado, Matthew P. Harrison, and Veronica Khauv, "Embryo Survival After Mifepristone: A Systematic Review of the Literature", *Issues in Law & Medicine* 32, no. 1 (2017): 3–18. (The article is available at stenoinstitute.org/resources.)

be injected; most doctors give 2 ml in each buttock. Some doctors instead will use the compounded 100 mg/ml formulation that requires a total volume of only 2 ml.

Besides the discomfort of shots, two other hurdles arose. Obtaining compounded medications had become increasingly difficult in many states due to additional regulations, perhaps in response to a series of spinal cord infections related to the injection of compounded medications (not progesterone) into the cerebral spinal fluid around the spinal cord. The other issue has been that the need for an injection could limit how soon a woman seeking APR could get her first dose.

When we were collecting data for the 2018 study, we had a meeting with some of the leaders of Obria Clinic in Orange County, California, because they were interested in improving and expanding their APR services. They mentioned that they had been tracking their own patients and had discovered that their reversal attempts were more successful after their medical director, E. Peter Anzaldo, MD, changed their protocol from injection to a high-dose oral protocol—a protocol we labeled the "high-dose oral" protocol in our paper. Our analysis confirmed that the group of women who received the high-dose oral protocol had a 68 percent successful reversal rate. After that, our favored recommended protocol was the high-dose protocol initiated by Dr. Anzaldo.

Then, in 2019, I visited Switzerland to give two talks to interested medical and pro-life professionals (see chapter 7). There, I met with Dr. Werner Foerster. Because the mifepristone dose used in Switzerland is 600 mg, instead of the 200 mg used in the United States, Dr. Foerster and others were using much higher doses of oral progesterone for APR. Their patients were tolerating the higher doses very well. After that and learning that doctors in the United

States were also safely using doses higher than the high-dose protocol, I and others increased our doses to 600 mg twice a day for two days, 400 mg twice a day for two days, then 400 mg at night until the end of the first trimester or for two weeks, whichever is longer.

More Science Made Simple

Clinical research on human beings will always be the most important evidence we can offer. However, basic science from research in test tubes and animals can be important in establishing foundations for what should be studied next and in filling knowledge gaps that are difficult to fill with research on humans.

I call the evidence supporting APR "the three pillars". The first pillar is our knowledge of how progesterone and mifepristone molecules compete for the same receptors. Early research by scientists at the US National Institutes of Health (NIH) demonstrated that increasing the concentration of progesterone in a test tube would negate the effects of mifepristone on cells cultured from human placentas.[8] That is exactly our APR strategy: administer supplemental progesterone to outcompete the mifepristone and win the battle at the receptor sites.

The second pillar is animal research. Early mifepristone studies were conducted on rats in Japan. They learned that when mifepristone was given alone to pregnant rats, all the embryos would be aborted. When progesterone was given at the same time as the mifepristone, far fewer

---

[8] Chandra Das and Kevin J. Catt, "Antifertility Actions of the Progesterone Antagonist RU 486 Include Direct Inhibition of Placental Hormone Secretion", *The Lancet* 330, no. 8559 (1987): 599–601, https://pubmed.ncbi.nlm.nih.gov/2887889/.

were aborted, demonstrating that the abortifacient effect of mifepristone was blunted by progesterone.[9] While this was important evidence, the experiments did not mirror real-life APR when a woman takes mifepristone first and progesterone later.

Stephen Sammut, PhD, a neuroscience researcher, developed another rat model of mifepristone abortion. Then he established a rat model of mifepristone reversal utilizing progesterone given subsequent to the mifepristone, simulating real-life APR.[10]

His elegant experiments showed that after mifepristone is administered to pregnant rats, characteristic changes occur, including bleeding in the vagina and a blunting of the normal pregnancy weight gain, all signifying that an abortion has begun. After the progesterone is given to the mother rats, bleeding stops, weight goes up, and the other changes induced by the mifepristone go away. Not only that, but the embryos also survive.[11] Dr. Sammut's research has shown that progesterone truly does reverse an abortion that has already started, rather than preventing it, thus confirming that abortion pill *reversal* is an apt term for what we do.

The US Food and Drug Administration (FDA) stated in its Pharmacology Review of mifepristone in the Drug Approval Packet, "Thus, the abortifacient activity of RU 486 is antagonized by progesterone allowing for normal pregnancy and delivery." This statement was a conclusion to

---

[9] S. Yamabe, K. Katayama, and M. Mochizuki, "The Effect of RU486 and Progesterone on Luteal Function During Pregnancy", *Nihon Naibunpi Gakkai Zasshi* 65, no. 5 (1989): 497–511, https://doi.org/10.1507/endocrine1927.65.5_497.

[10] Christina Camilleri and Stephen Sammut, "Progesterone-Mediated Reversal of Mifepristone-Induced Pregnancy Termination in a Rat Model: An Exploratory Investigation", *Scientific Reports* 13, no. 10942 (2023), https://www.nature.com/articles/s41598-023-38025-9. (The article is also available at stenoinstitute.org/resources.)

[11] Ibid.

studies done in rabbits showing that the rabbits that received progesterone with mifepristone had no abortions.[12] Thus, it seems that the FDA was prescient in anticipating APR.

The third pillar is composed of the studies in humans that we and others have completed, along with the more than 7,000 babies whose lives have been saved by APR. How can anyone see these beautiful faces and say that APR does not work or that pregnant women seeking to reverse their chemical abortions should not be given a second chance at choice?

---

[12] "Center for Drug Evaluation and Research Application Number: 20-687—Part 2," US Food and Drug Administration, accessed April 5, 2025, https://www.accessdata.fda.gov/drugsatfda_docs/nda/2000/20687_Mifepristone_phrmr_P2.pdf.

4

The Political Agenda That Got Mifepristone Approved

Just as Roussel Uclaf rushed to develop mifepristone, abortion proponents around the world hurried to get it approved in their respective countries in order to claim the "holy grail" that they had long sought—abortion at home with minimal input or support from medical professionals. The location of the abortion would shift from the abortion center to the woman's bathroom.

The World Health Organization (WHO) placed mifepristone and misoprostol on its list of "essential" medicines in 2005. The list includes many logical, life-saving choices such as penicillin and oxytocin (to induce labor and stop post-delivery bleeding). Many in the pro-life world wondered why abortion-causing drugs should be on the same list with the life-saving medications. How is abortion "life-saving"?

In the United States, abortion supporters, well connected to the Democratic Party, moved to have mifepristone approved. The FDA was designed as an apolitical organization whose sole purpose is protecting the American people from dangerous drugs and foods. Yet this was not the case when it came to the abortion pill. According to an in-depth article titled "Population Control, Chemical Abortion, and the Post-*Dobbs* Landscape" by Donna

Harrison, MD,[1] and court documents from an FDA lawsuit, the approval process for mifepristone was like that of no other drug.

In his first week in office in January 1993, President Bill Clinton directed his administration to approve chemical abortion in the United States. The Clinton administration then pressured Roussel Uclaf to grant the US rights to mifepristone to the Population Council—for free. After the Population Council received the rights to mifepristone, it submitted an investigational new drug (IND) application and worked closely with the FDA to ensure its approval. The FDA did not follow its own regulations in approving it. The drug had a favored status, and the rails were greased for its approval. The drug was approved on September 30, 2000, right before the highly contested presidential elections.[2]

The FDA was able to implement an accelerated approval process because it classified pregnancy as an illness instead of the normal physiologic reproductive process that it is and declared that chemical abortion provides a "meaningful therapeutic benefit".[3] In addition, the FDA never comprehensively studied the short- and long-term safety of mifepristone, in violation of the Food, Drug, and Cosmetic Act. The Pediatric Research Equity Act was violated because the effects on developing adolescent girls were never investigated. The drug was approved for use in children despite the lack of clinical trials that included children (those younger than age eighteen).[4]

---

[1] Donna Harrison, "Population Control, Chemical Abortion, and the Post-*Dobbs* Landscape", *Faith & Flourishing: A Journal of Karam Fellowship* 3 (2024), https://karamfellowship.org/ff-archive/.
[2] Ibid.
[3] Ibid.
[4] Ibid.

In the last several years, there has been great progress in requiring drugs that might be used in children to be tested in pediatric patients. The usual proponents of better research in children, such as the American Academy of Pediatrics, failed to object to the shortcuts the FDA allowed in the mifepristone approval process. Those shortcuts put girls' health and lives at risk.

Mifepristone was approved in the United States without a placebo-controlled, randomized trial, which violates the FDA regulations that require such a study before a new drug can be given approval. A placebo-controlled study is one in which one group of test subjects gets the drug being tested while the other group gets a placebo (a pill with no active ingredient). Randomized means that the subjects are assigned to one or the other group by a randomized process, usually computer generated.

The Spitz study, published in the prestigious *New England Journal of Medicine* in 1998 and used by the FDA to support the approval of mifepristone, was neither randomized nor placebo controlled.[5] The FDA used the loophole reserved for special life-saving drugs that can be approved without the stringent study requirements.[6] Of course, it begs the question, How is mifepristone life-saving either for the preborn baby or the mother?

Perhaps realizing it was compromising its reputation, the FDA instituted a Risk Evaluation and Mitigation Strategy (REMS), as it has done in the past with other dangerous drugs. The REMS required in-person dispensing and administration of mifepristone in a clinic setting. Special

---

[5] Irving M. Spitz, MD, DSc, C. Wayne Bardin, MD, Lauri Benton, MD, and Ann Robbins, PhD, "Early Pregnancy Termination with Mifepristone and Misoprostol in the United States", *New England Journal of Medicine* 338, no. 18 (1998): 1241–47, https://www.nejm.org/doi/full/10.1056/NEJM199804303381801.

[6] Harrison, "Population Control, Chemical Abortion".

registration was required for abortionists to become mifepristone prescribers. All complications and adverse reactions were required to be reported; however, an effective enforcement mechanism was not implemented.[7] In essence, experimentation occurred after the drug was approved.

Later Years

About two years after the approval of mifepristone abortion, plaintiffs represented by Alliance Defending Freedom, a public service law firm, filed a Citizen Petition to have the chemical abortion drug removed from the market because of the aforementioned irregularities in the approval process. In March 2016, fourteen years after the petition was filed, the FDA finally responded to and rejected the petition. The same day the petition was rejected, the FDA made changes affecting the safety and monitoring of mifepristone abortion. At that time, it extended the approval of the drug for use in an abortion up to ten weeks of pregnancy, up from the previous seven-week limit. Additionally, the required in-person visits were reduced from three to one. The requirement for abortionists and abortion centers to report complications, except deaths, was removed.[8] The ability of clinicians to conceal the complications of chemical abortions was now greater than ever.

In 2019, the favored status was again manifested. A generic version of mifepristone was approved without the usual studies required of generic drugs.[9]

---

[7] "NDA 20-687 Mifeprex (Mifepristone) Tablets, 200 mg: Risk Evaluation and Mitigation Strategy (REMS)", US FDA, accessed April 5, 2025, https://www.accessdata.fda.gov/drugsatfda_docs/rems/Mifeprex_2011-06-08_Full.pdf.

[8] Harrison, "Population Control, Chemical Abortion".

[9] Ibid.

In April 2021, early in President Joe Biden's tenure, the FDA issued a "nonenforcement decision" whereby the in-person, witnessed ingestion of mifepristone in a clinic would no longer be enforced. The new "nonenforcement" allowed mail-order procurement of mifepristone and misoprostol and was declared to be a temporary response to the COVID-19 pandemic public health emergency.[10]

A second Citizen Petition had been filed in 2019 asking the FDA to restore all the pre-2016 restrictions on mifepristone. This time, it took the FDA only two and a half years to respond to and reject the petition. On the same day in December 2021, the Biden administration approved the permanent right to send chemical abortion drugs through the mail.[11] As many suspected, the "temporary" "nonenforcement" during the COVID-19 pandemic was the proverbial camel getting his nose in the tent.

After the many frustrating years of stonewalling and delays by the FDA, in late 2022 Erik Baptist, the senior counsel of Alliance Defending Freedom, filed a lawsuit against the FDA in the United States District Court for the Northern District of Texas in Amarillo on behalf of Alliance for Hippocratic Medicine, American Association of Pro-Life Obstetricians and Gynecologists, American College of Pediatricians, Christian Medical & Dental Associations, and four individual doctors—Shaun Jester, DO; Regina Frost-Clark, MD; Tyler Johnson, DO; and me. The lawsuit raised all the concerns regarding the illegal approval of mifepristone as well as the relaxation of the REMS safety measures. Initially, the federal judge in Texas suspended the approval of mifepristone. However, an emergency appeal stayed the order. Eventually, the case

---

[10] Ibid.
[11] Ibid.

went to the US Supreme Court. The court ruled only on the legal standing that the plaintiffs had, not the merits of the case itself. Unfortunately, the high court ruled that none of the plaintiffs had legal standing to bring the lawsuit. However, several states have expressed interest in assuming the roles of plaintiffs and continuing the case.

We will need to stay tuned to see how this compelling case continues. Hopefully, the courts will force the FDA to play by its own rules and protect the health of all our citizens.

The unlevel playing field is not only in the federal arena. In 2023, the State of California sued Heartbeat International and RealOptions Obria Medical Clinics (of San Jose) asserting that by offering APR they are hurting women and providing misinformation. The Thomas More Society is defending Heartbeat and RealOptions.

Culture of Life Family Services, where I am medical director, has taken the offensive and sued the State of California. Represented by the law firm LiMandri & Jonna LLP, in conjunction with the Thomas More Society, we are asserting that by persecuting providers of APR life-saving treatment, the state is infringing on our free speech rights and our ability to practice medicine as we see best.

New York Attorney General Letitia James has sued Heartbeat International, CompassCare, and other providers of APR treatment in a case very similar to California's attack on APR providers. The Thomas More Society is also representing those plaintiffs and has filed suit against the attorney general in an effort to fend off the persecution.

The aggressive pro-abortion politics and abuse of the judicial system continue when those wedded to the pro-abortion agenda have power. However, those who support life have reason, truth, and expert legal eagles on their side.

5

The Growth of the Abortion Pill Industry

The mifepristone and misoprostol combination chemical abortion was developed in France and Switzerland and approved for clinical use in France and China in 1988. Approval was granted in 1991 in Great Britain and 1992 in Sweden. The drug was approved in Israel in 1999 and in the United States in 2000. By 2023, ninety-six countries had legalized the use of mifepristone and misoprostol for chemical abortion, according to the Guttmacher Institute.[1]

In 2014, about 30 percent of induced abortions in the United States were chemical abortions.[2] That percentage steadily increased so that by 2023, Guttmacher estimated that 63 percent of all US abortions were chemical.[3] The 2024 statistics are not yet available; however, reputable

---

[1] Gilda Sedgh and Irum Taqi, "Mifepristone for Abortion in a Global Context: Safe, Effective and Approved in Nearly 100 Countries", Policy Analysis, July 2023, Guttmacher Institute, accessed April 3, 2025, https://www.guttmacher.org/2023/07/mifepristone-abortion-global-context-safe-effective-and-approved-nearly-100-countries.

[2] Rachel K. Jones and Jenna Jerman, "Abortion Incidence and Service Availability in the United States, 2014", Perspectives on Sexual and Reproductive Health 49, no. 1 (2017), https://doi.org/10.1363/psrh.12015.

[3] "Monthly Abortion Provision Study", US Abortion Data Dashboard, Guttmacher Institute, accessed April 3, 2025, https://www.guttmacher.org/monthly-abortion-provision-study.

sources estimate that about 70 percent of all abortions in the United States are chemical abortions. We expect that percentage to increase as it has in other parts of the world. For example, according to the UK organization Abortion Rights, in 2022, 99 percent of all abortions in Scotland were chemical abortions.[4]

Planned Parenthood heavily promotes chemical abortion on its website, referring to it as "the abortion pill". The cost of a chemical abortion can vary, but $550 is a fair estimate. Meanwhile, a first-trimester surgical abortion will average about $600 at Planned Parenthood, according to a 2025 article on its website.[5]

There are several economic and strategic advantages for Planned Parenthood and other abortion providers to transition from surgical to chemical abortions. The biggest is that they will have to contract with far fewer expensive physician abortionists, who are aging and becoming more difficult to find. Stories abound of older abortionists making the circuit from one abortion center to the next, sometimes in different states.

It is clear that the vast majority of physicians do not want to perform abortions. According to a 2017 Guttmacher study, only 7 percent of private practice obstetrician gynecologists perform abortions.[6] A 2011 study by

---

[4] Alisa Berry Ryan, "Scottish Abortion Statistics 2022", May 31, 2023, Abortion Rights, accessed April 5, 2025, https://abortionrights.org.uk/scottish-abortion-statistics-2022/.

[5] "How Much Does an Abortion Cost?", Planned Parenthood, April 13, 2025, https://www.plannedparenthood.org/blog/how-much-does-an-abortion-cost#:~:text=Abortion%20pills%20(AKA%20medication%20abortion,can%20be%20between%20$1%2C500%2D2%2C000.

[6] "Most U.S. Obstetrician-Gynecologists in Private Practice Do Not Provide Abortions and Many Also Fail to Provide Referrals", News Release, November 27, 2017, Guttmacher Institute, https://www.guttmacher.org/news-release/2017/most-us-obstetrician-gynecologists-private-practice-do-not-provide-abortions.

researchers not affiliated with Guttmacher found that only 14 percent perform abortions.[7]

Although the reimbursement for chemical abortions is less than for surgical abortions, the associated overhead is much less. There are fewer procedure rooms, fewer supplies, fewer recovery rooms, less malpractice insurance, and fewer physician salaries. Additionally, the number of chemical abortions per day could be significantly higher than the number of surgical abortions per day.

According to Planned Parenthood's fiscal year 2022–2023 financial report, total revenue was $1.8 billion. Of that, $699 million came from government health services, reimbursements, and grants; that is, from our tax dollars.[8] Clearly Planned Parenthood is a big business; it is the backbone of Big Abortion, a critical part of the Medical-Abortion Complex.

Planned Parenthood has claimed that abortion services make up only a tiny part of its business. They rationalize that claim by counting every single encounter with a customer, client, or patient as a "service". Using that methodology, the 392,715 abortions conducted by Planned Parenthood in fiscal year 2022–2023 were only 4.3 percent of all services. However, looking at revenue generated, another picture emerges.

Assuming the average reimbursement for an abortion is $600, the total revenue for abortions in fiscal year 2022–2023 was $235.6 million. Total Planned Parenthood revenue

---

[7] Debra B. Stulberg, Annie M. Dude, Irma Dahlquist, and Farr A. Curlin, "Abortion Provision Among Practicing Obstetrician–Gynecologists", *Obstetrics & Gynecology* 118, no. 3 (2011): 609–14, https://doi.org/10.1097/AOG.0b013e31822ad973.

[8] "Above and Beyond: Annual Report 2022–2023", Planned Parenthood, accessed April 5, 2025, https://www.plannedparenthood.org/uploads/filer_public/ce/f6/cef6efdb-919a-4211-bb5c-ce0d61fda7f5/2024-ppfa-annual report-c3-digital.pdf.

minus private contributions was $1.05 billion. Therefore, 22 percent of Planned Parenthood's business-generated revenue came from abortion. That figure, 22 percent, is much more than the "tiny" figure of 4.3 percent that Planned Parenthood reports.

The numbers are growing too. According to the Charlotte Lozier Institute's April 2024 Planned Parenthood Fact Sheet, the number of abortions in 2023 increased by 5 percent since the previous year and 20 percent in the last ten years.[9]

That report reveals that abortions by Planned Parenthood have been increasing since 2017. The increase in the first fiscal year after the 2022 *Dobbs v. Jackson* decision, which overturned *Roe v. Wade*, shows that although documented abortions fell drastically in states with strong pro-life laws, abortions in the United States were on the rise overall. According to Guttmacher, in 2023, 1.034 million abortions were performed, an 11 percent increase compared to 2020.[10]

The number of telehealth and mail-order abortions has been increasing too. This is due in large part to the Biden administration's relaxation of the in-person requirements for obtaining mifepristone and misoprostol.

It is important to clarify here what I mean by the terms *telehealth* and *mail-order abortions*. A telehealth abortion is when a pregnant woman seeking an abortion has a virtual visit via an audio-video platform like Zoom. The woman shows the medical practitioner her pregnancy test and discusses the details of a chemical abortion. The abortion pills

---

[9] "Fact Sheet: Planned Parenthood's 2022-23 Annual Report", April 17, 2024, Charlotte Lozier Institute, https://lozierinstitute.org/fact-sheet-planned-parenthoods-2022-23-annual-report/.

[10] "Monthly Abortion Provision Study", US Abortion Data Dashboard, Guttmacher Institute, accessed April 5, 2025, https://www.guttmacher.org/monthly-abortion-provision-study.

are then sent via the mail. A mail-order abortion is similar except there is no virtual medical visit. Instead, the person ordering the abortion pills—who, by the way, could be a man—simply completes an online questionnaire and then obtains the drugs through the mail.

The relaxation of the in-person requirement occurred during the public health emergency surrounding COVID-19. If this accommodation had truly been because of the COVID-19 pandemic, once the emergency passed, the restriction would have been reinstated. It has not been.

That and a growing online market for mifepristone and misoprostol has led to the "Wild West" of abortion. Women's health and safety have been sacrificed for the sake of ideology and profit.

The US Government's Role in the Development of the Medical-Abortion Complex

Donna Harrison, MD, wrote an insightful and comprehensive paper in *Faith & Fellowship* in 2024.[11] She connected the dots between the population control movement in the 1930s to the *Roe v. Wade* decision to the approval and promotion of mifepristone abortion, all aided and abetted by the US government.

In the 1930s, the Rockefeller Foundation funded the Office of Population Research at Princeton University. In 1952, John D. Rockefeller convened a meeting of influential leaders that led to the creation of the Population Council. The Rockefeller, Carnegie, and other well-endowed

---

[11] Donna Harrison, "Population Control, Chemical Abortion, and the Post-*Dobbs* Landscape", *Faith & Flourishing: A Journal of Karam Fellowship* 3 (2024), https://karamfellowship.org/ff-archive/.

foundations poured money into the Population Council in order to find ways to limit or decrease human population, assuming that "overpopulation" would eventually ruin the planet.

In 1969, the government created the Commission on Population Growth and the American Future. A few years later, John D. Rockefeller authored its first report, which stated, "No substantial benefits will result from further growth of the Nation's population."[12] Rockefeller called for the legalization of abortion throughout the land. The report was issued just before the landmark *Roe v. Wade* decision that made abortion a constitutional right.

In interviews given in 2009 and 2012, the late Justice Ruth Bader Ginsburg, a staunch supporter of abortion, acknowledged the connection between population fears and the legalization of abortion: "Frankly I had thought that at the time *Roe* was decided, there was concern about population growth and particularly growth in populations that we don't want to have too many of. So that *Roe* was going to be then set up for Medicaid funding for abortion."[13] Medicaid funds abortions only for poor women. The population control envisioned was one rooted in eugenics. While Black people make up about 13 percent of the US population, around 39 percent of abortions are performed on Black women. Planned Parenthood's Susan A. Cohen wrote in 2008, "This much is true: In the United States, the abortion rate for black women is almost five times that for white women."[14]

The Population Council funded research by Dr. Étienne-Émile Baulieu and the large pharmaceutical corporation

---

[12] Ibid.

[13] Ibid.

[14] Susan A. Cohen, "Abortion and Women of Color: The Bigger Picture", *Guttmacher Policy Review* 11, no. 3 (2008), https://www.guttmacher.org/gpr/2008/08/abortion-and-women-color-bigger-picture.

Roussel Uclaf in France that led to the development of RU-486, later called mifepristone. The Council, in turn, received its funding from two government agencies, the United States Agency for International Development (USAID) and the National Institute of Child Health and Development (NICHD), a branch of the National Institutes of Health (NIH).[15] In 2025, USAID is in the crosshairs of the second Trump administration's Department of Government Efficiency. Besides USAID's role in promoting abortion, there are serious allegations of fraud, abuse, and having funded left-wing organizations.

The Risks Associated with Telehealth and Mail-Order Abortions

There are several risks women take when they embark on mail-order or telehealth abortions. The most potentially catastrophic is an undiagnosed ectopic pregnancy.

Fertilization—when the sperm and egg cells unite to create a new human individual—occurs in the fallopian tube. An ectopic pregnancy is when the early embryo does not make it to the uterus but instead implants in another location, the most common being the wall of the fallopian tube. As that preborn baby grows, the tube is stretched until it ruptures. A ruptured tube will bleed profusely and place the mother's life at risk. Although 1 to 2 percent of all pregnancies in the United States are ectopic pregnancies,[16] generally a woman receives treatment before serious bleeding has occurred.

---

[15] Harrison, "Population Control, Chemical Abortion".

[16] Laura M. Mann, Kristen Kreisel, Eloisa Llata, Jaeyoung Hong, and Elizabeth A. Torrone, "Trends in Ectopic Pregnancy Diagnoses in United States Emergency Departments, 2006–2013", *Maternal and Child Health Journal* 24, no. 2 (2020): 213–21, https://doi.org/10.1007/s10995-019-02842-0.

Women undergoing telehealth or mail-order abortions will often not have ultrasounds, as they would have had they gone to an abortion center. Without an ultrasound, a woman will not know if she has an ectopic pregnancy. Once at home, when bleeding starts in her bathroom, she likely will attribute heavy bleeding to the chemical abortion process, since she was told that she will bleed. As the bleeding continues, she may lose consciousness and be unable to call for emergency help. She may die on her bathroom floor.

Another risk of telehealth and mail-order abortions is Rh sensitization. About 15 percent of the US population is Rh negative with regard to blood type.[17] If a patient with Rh-negative blood receives a transfusion with Rh-positive blood, the recipient's immune system will recognize the Rh protein on the Rh-positive blood cells as foreign; an immune response attacking the donor red blood cells will ensue. During pregnancy, delivery, miscarriages, and abortions, there is some mixture of blood between the baby and the mother. If an Rh-negative mother carries an Rh-positive baby, there will be a risk that her immune system will be alerted to the foreign Rh protein. The immune exposure will lead to the production of Rh-specific antibodies and T-cells that will attack the Rh-positive blood cells. The blood cells that are attacked will be destroyed, leading to fetal anemia and sometimes fetal heart failure. As part of routine prenatal care, we test all pregnant mothers, and those who are Rh negative get a shot of Rh immune globulin (brand name RhoGam). The Rh immune globulin blankets the Rh protein so that the mother's immune system never sees the foreign

---

[17] "The Significance of Being Rh Negative or Rh Positive", May 1, 2016, Carter BloodCare, https://www.carterbloodcare.org/blog/blog/2016/05/the-significance-of-being-rh-negative-or-rh-positive/; "Practice Bulletin No. 181: Prevention of Rh D Alloimmunization", *Obstetrics & Gynecology* 130, no. 2 (2017): e57–e70, https://doi.org/10.1097/AOG.0000000000002232.

protein and thus is not activated. The strategy of testing for Rh and treating Rh negative mothers has led to a 90 percent decrease in maternal antibodies against Rh.[18]

Up until very recently, the standard at abortion centers was to test women who were having abortions and administer a shot of Rh immune globulin to those who were negative. With telehealth and mail-order abortions, the 15 percent of women who are Rh negative may never know it and certainly will not receive the Rh immune globulin. This is important because once the immune system detects the Rh protein, it never forgets it. Once sensitized, an Rh-negative woman will be at risk for severe complications, including stillbirths, in all future wanted pregnancies with Rh-positive preborn babies.[19] It is like a curse that cannot be undone.

Why did the American College of Obstetricians and Gynecologists (ACOG) change the recommendation of checking Rh status at the time of abortions? Their stated reason in the 2024 clinical update was that the risk of Rh sensitization is low in first-trimester abortions. The clinical update cited two newer studies, one with only 37 patients and one with 506. The statement declared, "The study authors acknowledge that a main limitation of their study is that the true fetal–maternal hemorrhage volume necessary to trigger Rh sensitization remains unknown."[20] In other words, changes were made to longstanding recommendations based on assumptions and opinion. It is an interesting coincidence that this change in policy occurred at the time of increasing telehealth and mail-order abortions.

---

[18] "Practice Bulletin No. 181".
[19] Ibid.
[20] "ACOG Clinical Practice Update: Rh D Immune Globulin Administration After Abortion or Pregnancy Loss at Less Than 12 Weeks of Gestation", *Obstetrics & Gynecology* 144, no. 6 (2024): e140–e143, https://doi.org/10.1097/AOG.0000000000005733.

Lack of an ultrasound may lead to misdating of a pregnancy; a woman may take mifepristone past ten weeks, when it is less effective at ending the pregnancy. It is interesting and contradictory that the ACOG recommends routine ultrasound as part of prenatal care partly because women often cannot remember the first day of their last menstrual period.[21] However, when it comes to chemical abortion, they say that ultrasound is not needed routinely.[22] Lack of an ultrasound or a confirmatory pregnancy test may lead to nonpregnant women, who have misinterpreted home pregnancy tests, taking mifepristone. Such scenarios have not been studied and likely never will be.

Other risks that are sure to increase with the rise of telehealth and mail-order abortions include misdiagnosis and delayed diagnosis of infections and serious bleeding. Delays in treatment of these complications could lead to catastrophic consequences.

Besides the medical risks, there are important social risks to women. Who is to say that next to a woman accessing a telehealth abortion there is not a man seated nearby, off camera, who is coercing her? Additionally, a man could easily pretend to be a woman and use a mail-order website to buy mifepristone and misoprostol. I know of at least one case in which a partner added mifepristone to a pregnant woman's drink—without her knowledge—in order to abort his preborn child.

Antonio Marchi of Right to Life Michiana reported during his speech at his organization's 2024 fundraiser that

---

[21] "Practice Bulletin No. 175: Ultrasound in Pregnancy", *Obstetrics & Gynecology* 128, no. 6 (2016): e241–e256, https://doi.org/10.1097/AOG.0000000000001815.

[22] "Medical Abortion up to 70 Days of Pregnancy", ACOG Practice Bulletin 225, October 2020, https://www.acog.org/clinical/clinical-guidance/practice-bulletin/articles/2020/10/medication-abortion-up-to-70-days-of-gestation.

it took him only fifteen seconds on an online site to get to the point where he could pay for abortion drugs. I visited the Plan C website, and within several clicks, I was at a menu of six online vendors that sell mifepristone and misoprostol to "all ages". No online consultation with a medical practitioner is required. All indicate you can get pills in advance; pills can be sold to men and women and minors since there is no way to verify sex or age.[23]

The Your Safe Abortion website has a page that allows people to purchase abortion pills from Switzerland. It states, "According to our extensive experience, where abortions are officially prohibited, our Abortion kits pass customs without problems in most countries. For recipients in the European Union, we ship from an EU country; for recipients in the United States or Canada, we ship from the United States. In those few cases where customs does hold the parcel, we send a replacement for free." The available kits include Abortion Pill Kit, AntiPreg Kit, Mifepristone Misoprostol combipack, and Cytolog (which contains only misoprostol, not mifepristone).[24]

An investigative report by American Life League (ALL) in 2024 discovered a network of individuals and organizations that ALL dubbed a cartel. The "community" groups import abortion pills from foreign countries and then distribute them in the United States, violating or circumventing US laws.[25] One such group was Las Libres, which is based in Mexico and had a page on the Plan C website in 2024. All a person needed in order to obtain abortion

---

[23] Plan C, accessed April 5, 2025, https://www.plancpills.org/.

[24] "Buy Abortion Pills in Switzerland", Your Safe Abortion, accessed April 5, 2025, https://your-safe-abortion.com/countries/buy-mtp-pills-in-switzerland/.

[25] "Beneath the Surface: Exposing the Abortion Pill Drug Cartel", American Life League, September 2024, https://www.all.org/wp-content/uploads/2024/09/ALL_AbortionPillReport2024.pdf.

drugs was a first name and a date of the last menstrual period, neither of which is verifiable by the provider. In early 2025, Las Libres was no longer on the Plan C website; instead, the Las Libres link redirected the user to a group called DASH.[26]

An NPR article by Elissa Nadworny spotlighted Massachusetts Medication Abortion Access Project (MAP), run by Angel Foster, MD, PhD. According to Nadworny, "The MAP is one of just four groups in the US sending pills to people who live in states that ban or restrict abortion. They can do this because they are in states that have passed shield laws that protect them legally. Eight states have such laws. Medication sent by shield law providers now accounts for about 10 percent of abortions nationwide—as many as 12,000 a month."[27]

The ALL report listed three examples of known instances of coerced or forced attempted abortions. CBS reported that a Texas man surreptitiously gave his pregnant wife misoprostol (the second drug in the mifepristone-misoprostol protocol) to induce abortion. The baby girl survived but has had complications related to her preterm birth. That man was sentenced to 180 days in jail.[28]

In 2023, a Florida woman tried to bribe her ex-boyfriend so that he would give his pregnant current girlfriend an

---

[26] "The Plan C Guide to Abortion Pills by Mail: Information About Abortion Pills from DASH", Plan C, accessed April 12, 2025, https://www.plancpills.org/dash.

[27] Elissa Nadworny, "Inside a Medical Practice Sending Abortion Pills to States Where They're Banned", NPR, August 7, 2024, https://www.npr.org/2024/08/06/nx-s1-5037750/abortion-pills-bans-telehealth-mail-mifepristone-misoprostol.

[28] "Texas Man Gets Jail Time for Drugging Wife's Drinks to Induce an Abortion", CBS News Texas, February 10, 2024, https://www.cbsnews.com/texas/news/texas-man-gets-jail-time-for-drugging-wifes-drinks-to-induce-an-abortion/.

abortion pill. He reported her to law enforcement. She admitted "she got the pill from a virtual doctor online and knew it was an abortion pill." She offered to pay the would-be hit man with AirPods.[29]

In May 2024, a man in Massachusetts was arrested after giving the woman he was dating misoprostol pills, telling her they were iron pills or vitamins. The preborn baby died.[30]

The low bar for procuring abortions via telehealth or mail order will continue to fuel the growth of this industry, and these will become the tools of rapists, child molesters, and sex traffickers. Ideology and profit have trumped common sense and the protection of vulnerable women.

The Deliberate Blurring of the Lines

The Medical-Abortion Complex knows its flagship product, abortion, is inherently unattractive to most people. A Gallup poll in 2024 found that only 35 percent of Americans favor legal abortion "under any circumstances".[31]

Contraception, on the other hand, is well accepted by most Americans. Now the Medical-Abortion Complex is seeking to blur the lines between the two. The effect will be to desensitize people to abortion and create a safe market for mifepristone and other abortifacients that will be protected, even if abortion were to be banned in all states.

---

[29] "HCSO: Woman Accused of Trying to Get Father of Unborn Child to Give Abortion Pill to Pregnant Mother", Fox News Tampa Bay, June 2, 2023, https://www.fox13news.com/news/hcso-woman-tries-to-pay-father-to-kill-his-unborn-child-with-airpods.

[30] Christina Hager, "Massachusetts Man Accused of Secretly Giving Girlfriend Abortion Pill to End Pregnancy", WBZ CBS News, updated May 29, 2024, https://www.cbsnews.com/boston/news/abortion-pill-misoprostol-boyfriend-arrested-pregnant-girlfriend/.

[31] "Abortion", Gallup, accessed April 5, 2025, https://news.gallup.com/poll/1576/abortion.aspx.

An article by Carrie N. Baker titled "Mifepristone as Weekly Contraception Performs 'Beyond Expectations' in Clinical Trials" highlights the work of Dr. Rebecca Gomperts, the founder of Women on Waves, an organization that seeks to circumvent sovereign nations' laws by bringing abortion by mail or sea. She was one of the organizers of a study of 550 women in Moldova, a small Eastern European nation of fewer than three million people, that evaluated mifepristone given once weekly as a contraceptive. "'There has never been a clear distinction between contraception and abortion,' said Gomperts, noting that people disagree about when pregnancy starts—at fertilization, implantation or beyond", the article stated.[32] That's exactly the message they want to spread: confusion on when a human being comes into existence. This message is in direct conflict with the science of embryology: An individual human being begins when sperm and egg unite at fertilization.

---

[32] Carrie N. Baker, "Mifepristone as Weekly Contraceptive Performs 'Beyond Expectations' in Clinical Trials", *Ms. Magazine*, January 7, 2025, https://msmagazine.com/2025/01/07/mifepristone-weekly-contraceptive-clinical-trials-abortion-pill-birth-control/.

6

Reversal in the United States

We have seen tremendous growth in the abortion pill reversal movement since its humble beginnings with the two parallel cases of Dr. Matthew Harrison in 2006 and Dr. Jonnalyn Belocura and me in 2008. I call it a movement because that is exactly what it has been. It has been a coalescence of the goodwill, innovation, compassion, and commitment of a growing number of health-care professionals and other talented individuals. The movement has always focused on the woman and her preborn child, offering that mother a second chance at choice, if she desires it.

That spirit of proposing but never imposing has never weakened. Many of the women I have met who have taken mifepristone and considered reversal have expressed great gratitude, whether they have chosen to reverse or not.

That spirit has also led to the organic and steady growth of the program. APR is so prevalent now that not all reversal cases come through the Abortion Pill Rescue Network run by Heartbeat International. Heartbeat estimates that as of June 2025, more than 7,000 preborn babies have been saved by APR, and there are over 1,400 doctors, other medical professionals, and clinics in the network. Women have been helped in all 50 states and in more than 93 countries.

The people at Heartbeat foresaw the promise of APR and how it could become a pro-life game changer. When Culture of Life Family Services sought a new home for the

APR program, it was a smooth negotiation process. I knew that when we sold the program—for one dollar!—it would be in good hands. As one of our supporters quipped, our APR baby had grown up.

Key players at Heartbeat who have facilitated APR's growth include the president, Jor-El Godsey; Christa Brown, RN, who has led the program since 2018; chairperson of the board, Peggy Hartshorn; attorney Danielle White; Lisa Searle, RN; Brooke Myrick, RN; Teresa Tholany, RN; Kelly McCallister, RN; Ashley Vance, RN; Brent Boles, MD; twenty-five hotline nurses; and others. Their compassion, commitment, and diligence have grown the APR Network into a world-class organization.

Besides Dr. Matthew Harrison and Dr. Mary Davenport, there have been many other courageous and compassionate APR physician champions. The American Association of Pro-Life Obstetricians and Gynecologists (AAPLOG), arguably the most influential pro-life medical group in the world, recognized the promise of APR as early as 2012. Dr. Davenport recommended that I be elected to the AAPLOG board, and I became the first family physician to serve on that board.

Joseph DeCook, MD, was president at that time and was very supportive. Allan Sawyer, MD, followed Dr. DeCook and moved full steam ahead. Donna Harrison, MD, was a mifepristone expert long before I helped develop APR. Her support and insight have been invaluable. Christina Francis, MD, the current president of AAPLOG, has been a strong, clear, and coherent voice for APR and the protection of women and their preborn babies, in general. Numerous board members at AAPLOG have been and continue to be very supportive of our mission.

Outside of AAPLOG and Heartbeat, several physicians have been and continue to be tireless champions. Many drop everything to take calls, see patients after hours, meet them at emergency departments, and even arrange transportation when none is available. I have been impressed and infinitely blessed to witness the compassion, empathy, professionalism, selflessness, courage, and competence of APR doctors and other practitioners who truly are my heroes.

Knowing that I am leaving out some stellar doctors, I want to highlight several. Karen Poehailos, MD, of My Catholic Doctor has been a tireless advocate for women in difficult pregnancies in many roles and many states. William Lile, MD, of ProLife Doc in Florida is a passionate speaker and hard-hitting educator on APR and pro-life topics. Paddy Jim Baggot, MD, in Los Angeles has been innovative and totally committed to maximizing patients' chances for successful reversals. Sister Dede Byrne, MD, and Marguerite Duane, MD, have been a dynamic duo serving APR patients in our nation's capital. Manrique Iriarte, MD, performed the first reversal of methotrexate, a drug that is not commonly used for chemical abortions. The championing of APR by Rolando De Leon, MD, led to many physicians in South Florida following suit. Lloyd Pierre, MD, and Angelina Giles, DNP, of Sancta Familia Medical Clinic in Omaha have developed a new protocol that will be published in an upcoming medical article. Kathleen Raviele, MD; Monique Ruberu, MD; William Toffler, MD; and many more have been very committed in bringing APR to their communities. Many APR doctors risked their professional reputations, bucking the American College of Obstetricians and Gynecologists (ACOG) party line by endorsing, supporting, and promoting APR (see chapter 26 on big medicine's opposition to APR).

Nonmedical people have been an important part of the movement too. Paul DeBeasi published a well-received review article on APR science in *The Linacre Quarterly*, the peer-reviewed journal of the Catholic Medical Association.[1] He also established and maintains a website that catalogs all the research around APR.[2]

APR is strong and growing in the United States and around the world. More women than ever are seeking a second chance at choice because more than ever have heard of it. Most pregnancy help centers now know of APR and support it in some way. Increasing numbers of emergency medicine doctors have heard of it. Whether the ACOG likes it or not, its relentless criticism of and attacks against APR have made it a familiar term to obstetricians; as the saying goes, any publicity is good publicity.

Slowly but surely, APR will become the standard of care. My goal is that in the future, a woman seeking a second chance at choice will simply call her primary physician or ob-gyn or visit the nearest emergency department to start the reversal process. It is safe and effective. It does not need to be complicated.

---

[1] Paul L.C. DeBeasi, "Mifepristone Antagonization with Progesterone to Avert Medication Abortion: A Scoping Review," *Linacre Quarterly* 90, no. 4 (2003): 395–407, https://doi.org/10.1177/00243639231176592.

[2] "APR Science", accessed April 12, 2025, https://aprscience.org/.

7

It's a Small World

Abortion pill reversal has spread to numerous countries besides the United States. Women who change their minds would like the opportunity of a second chance at choice. In most countries, as in the United States, APR started with one woman who had started her chemical abortion and made a phone call asking for help.

Australia

Debbie Garratt, RN, from the University of Notre Dame School of Nursing in Sydney, Australia, met me when I gave the keynote address at the national Right to Life League conference in New Orleans in the summer of 2015. In August, she reached out to Debbie Bradel, RN, our APR nurse manager, inquiring about APR. Eventually, I began to correspond with her and Dr. Joseph Turner, also of Australia.

Since February of that year, Debbie Bradel had been corresponding with Carolyn Morgan from Canberra to help her and others start APR in Australia. Carolyn had been working with Dr. Terrence Kent. Apparently, Carolyn and Debbie Garratt had been unaware of each other's efforts.

After the group started an Australian mifepristone reversal network, Australian authorities put the brakes on APR down under. Treatment was allowed only as part of research protocols. With those limitations, Dr. Turner began a multistep process of developing more research protocols to test the safety and effectiveness of APR. Thus far, Dr. Turner, Debbie Garratt, and their colleagues have published at least three articles in peer-reviewed medical literature.

Mexico

I was invited to give talks at two universities in Mexico in 2016. The talks were well attended and enthusiastically received. The main champions were two physicians, Dr. Pilar Calva and Dr. Angela Monarres. I was also able to meet with some people who were running a pro-life pregnancy help line for women in crisis. I thought that the established hotline would be ideal to serve as a Spanish-language APR hotline, not only for Mexico but for all of Latin America. For reasons never clear to me, that adaptation never came to fruition. However, a new group is organizing an APR network, and they have invited me to speak at a conference for doctors in Mexico.

Russia

In 2017, I received the following email:

> Dear colleagues,
> My name is Alexey and I am your colleague, a MD from Russia. We have about a million RU-486 abortions

in Russia annually and the number of cases when a woman changes her mind is very high.

We have found your APR technique in 2015, translated and posted it in Russian internet. Recently we have started to receive positive feedbacks from women who saved their children after progesterone injections.

So I would like to express our deepest gratitude for your splendid work and wish you success in saving lives.

Here is the link to our APR website: http://ru-486.ru/kak-ostanovit-medabort/.

All the best,
Dr. Alexey Fokin

I was thrilled to receive this message from a Russian doctor whom I did not know. I did know that as a result of Communism, abortion had been forced on Russians and had become extremely common. Due to prevalent abortion, widespread contraception use, and other factors, by the early 2000s Russia—not unlike other European countries—was facing a demographic winter. Their births were not keeping up with their deaths, and their population was aging very quickly.

Even after the collapse of Communism, abortion was still engrained in the culture, but more Russians and their leaders were realizing the negative societal and demographic consequences of abortion. It was in this changing political and social tide that Dr. Fokin introduced APR. Over the years, Dr. Fokin and I have continued our correspondence, and he has made strategic connections in the medical community in order to spread the good news of APR. He is currently conducting APR research in Russia.

In 2022, I learned from Dr. Fokin that the leading gynecologic institute in Russia had recommended giving progesterone to women who wished to reverse their mifepristone abortions. That proclamation carried the weight of what we call "standard of care", which is what any patient in a particular situation may be offered as treatment.

Furthermore, on June 4, 2024, the Russian Ministry of Health proclaimed that abortion pill reversal should be offered to women seeking to stop their mifepristone abortions. The following is an English translation of the Ministry of Health guidance, provided by Dr. Fokin:

> This year, on June 7, 2024, the Ministry of Health approved new clinical guidelines for obstetricians and gynecologists. Here they are:
> Basic recommendations for stopping medical abortion:
> 1. To stop a medical abortion, the patient's written consent is required.
> 2. Recommended regimens according to the instructions for indication, prevention, and treatment of threatened and incipient miscarriage.
> 3. Progesterone can be administered intramuscularly, orally, or topically.
> 4. Ultrasound control is required!

While in Western countries medical societies and governments are placing obstacles in the way of APR, in Russia APR is recognized and sanctioned by organized medicine and the government. I am quite impressed that the movement Dr. Fokin started is bearing such fruit. Dr. Fokin's network now receives about twenty to thirty-five calls per month, mostly from women in Russia, Kazakhstan, and Uzbekistan. He estimates that twelve to twenty per month start progesterone. He and his colleagues have helped many hundreds of women seeking a second chance at choice.

On September 23, 2023, via teleconference, I presented a talk on APR in English that was interpreted into Russian for a large conference on abortion and women's health held in Moscow for medical, pro-life, and religious leaders. There were over three hundred attendees; later Dr. Fokin told me the talk was well received. I had already been booked to give a talk at St. Mary Byzantine Catholic Church in Marblehead, Ohio, that day, and while I was waiting to give my in-person talk in Ohio, I found a room with a table from which I could deliver my talk to the folks in Russia. Some of the people setting up lunch for the Ohio conference could be seen in the background during my presentation. It was a busy and fruitful day.

Switzerland

I met Dominik Müggler-Schwager and some of his associates the evening before the March for Life in Washington, D.C., in January 2019. During the meeting, Dominik explained to me how he and others wanted to add APR to their life-affirming mission. Dominik is the head of Schweizerische Hilfe für Mutter und Kind (SHMK), which translates in English as Swiss Aid for Mother and Child. He left a successful career in corporate Switzerland to begin SHMK, which provides material and spiritual assistance to women in crisis pregnancies.

By 2019, they had started an innovative baby rescue service for women in crisis. At certain hospitals, they had paid for the installation of a baby window, which was accessible from the outside. A mother who could not care for her baby could anonymously open the window, place the baby in the bassinet, close the window, ring the bell, and leave, confident that her baby would receive immediate attention and eventually be adopted into a loving family. The hope was that this could be an option for those who might otherwise abort their babies or abandon them after birth.

At the meeting, Dominik invited me to go to Switzerland to give talks on APR to both medical personnel and pro-life staff members. We began making preparations for the summer visit. In June 2019, Liz and I traveled to Switzerland, first to Bern, then to Basel. I gave a talk at the University of Bern to a largely medical audience. They were very receptive to the information and data that I presented, including the findings of our 2018 APR study. All in that community were not so welcoming, however. Outside the lecture hall on the sidewalk, some protesters had scrawled negative messages, including one in clear English: "Dr. Delgado, go home."

The talk I gave the next day in Basel was mostly to workers from pregnancy help centers like SHMK. They were people in the trenches, more interested in the logistics of starting an APR program.

Later that second day, we got to spend the night at the home of Dr. and Mrs. Werner Foerster in Einsiedeln. Dr. Foerster was the unofficial medical director of the Swiss APR efforts. Because in Switzerland they were using 600 mg of mifepristone—as opposed to the 200 mg in the United States—for chemical abortion, he was utilizing higher doses of progesterone, safely and successfully. It was because of Dr. Foerster's use of higher progesterone doses as well as some American doctors using higher doses that I later started using 600 mg doses twice a day for the first two days of APR therapy.

The implementation of an APR network has been an uphill battle. While the Swiss federal government allows the provision of mifepristone and misoprostol without a doctor's visit or prescription, the regulations demand that APR be initiated only after a physician visit, another double standard.[1]

The United Kingdom and the Republic of Ireland

Dr. Dermot Kearney, an Irishman living in England, is a true hero. He has been persecuted as much as anyone because of his relentless efforts to give women a second chance at choice (see his story in chapter 23).

Dr. Kearney is a cardiologist by training who decided he needed to help pregnant women in Great Britain who were seeking to reverse their chemical abortions. His medical license was suspended because of his courage and perseverance. Eventually, his license was restored, and he was vindicated.

Doctors in Ireland have similarly been targeted. The Irish situation is somewhat ironic, since until 2018 Ireland was one of the most pro-life countries in the world. Pro-abortion activists and government officials effectively devised a strategy that many felt deceived the public. The result was that the electorate approved a referendum that repealed Amendment Eight of the Irish Constitution, thus legalizing abortion in Ireland.[2]

With the tide turned, abortion pill reversal was aggressively attacked. An Irish physician has a case pending with

---

[1] The Swiss APR website is https://www.rettet-mein-baby.ch/.

[2] Brian Lawless, "Ireland Votes to Repeal the 8th Amendment in Historic Abortion Referendum—And Marks a Huge Cultural Shift", *The Conversation*, May 26, 2018, https://theconversation.com/ireland-votes-to-repeal-the-8th-amendment-in-historic-abortion-referendum-and-marks-a-huge-cultural-shift-97297.

the Irish medical council because he provided life-saving APR to a woman who wanted a second chance at choice. There is a joint effort in the United Kingdom and Ireland to educate the public in both countries about APR.[3]

Canada

In 2020, Alliance for Life Ontario invited me to give a talk on APR. Doctors and other supporters of APR have been battling Canadian medical societies and the government-provided socialized medical system for years. Although the resistance is less than in the United Kingdom and Ireland, it has been difficult, nonetheless. Every country has its own version of the Medical-Abortion Complex. Canada also has its own APR network.[4]

Lithuania

Dr. Richard Cervin, a physician in Lithuania, reached out to me in 2022 inquiring about APR. In an email, he enthusiastically stated, "The statistics of your successes are of course to be doubled (at least!): to include also the mothers themselves to whom you bring back (lifelong) joy of having the child and saving them from the complications of chemical abortion!"

Dr. Cervin, gynecologist Dr. Virgilijus Rudzinskas, and others have been champions of APR in that Baltic country, with assistance from the Catholic Church. Since 2023,

---

[3] Their website is abortionpillreversal.ie.
[4] This network's website is abortionpillreversal.ca. The website has a chat feature as well as a toll-free telephone number.

the abortion pill has been legal in Lithuania, up to nine weeks of pregnancy.

Colombia

Colombia has a special place in my heart since it was there that my parents and five older brothers were born and lived until they emigrated to the United States, where I was born. I still have many cousins in that beautiful country. It was not until 2006 that abortion was made legal under certain narrow circumstances. In 2022, abortion was fully legalized up to twenty-four weeks of pregnancy by decree of the Constitutional Court (sounds like the United States Supreme Court's *Roe v. Wade* ruling).

During the COVID-19 pandemic in 2020–2021, abortion supporters took advantage of the situation, much like what happened in the United States, and heavily promoted and facilitated chemical abortion. A group, ironically called Profamilia, is the biggest supporter of abortion in the country and created a website where a chemical abortion kit could be obtained.

In March 2023, I presented my first webinar in Spanish on APR. The webinar was cosponsored by Heartbeat International and a Colombian organization called Fundación Amor y Vida (Love and Life Foundation) and was titled "*Revetir el aborto quimico es posible!*" ("Reversal of chemical abortion is possible!"). In Spanish, APR can be translated as RAQ, for *reversion del aborto quimico*. Anamaria Vargas, the strategy chief of Fundación Amor y Vida, told us the webinar was well received and many in the community had requested a recording of it.

According to Anamaria, many health professionals are afraid they will lose their jobs if they offer pro-life alternatives, including APR, to pregnant women considering abortion. The webinar was a big step in the encouragement and education of health-care professionals in Colombia and other Latin American countries.

Other Countries

According to Dr. Janez Rifel, there are about three thousand abortions per year in Slovenia, and the percentage of chemical abortions is rising, as in other countries. In 2011, a pro-life institute called Institute ŽIV!M (I Live) was started to help women in crisis pregnancies. In May 2021, the first woman seeking reversal reached out to the institute. In 2024, a family doctor joined Dr. Rifel and others to establish a Slovenian emergency hotline.[5]

Israel has had at least one APR case. The nonprofit pro-life group Be'ad Chaim helped connect a woman seeking reversal to a doctor in Israel. According to Sandy Shoshani, the executive director of Be'ad Chaim, a common saying of rabbis is "When you save one life, it is as though you have saved the world."[6]

Europe, of course, considers itself to be a liberal, progressive stalwart. When it comes to APR, the Medical-Abortion Complex is anything but liberal, inclusive, or diverse. It is their way or the highway—and they have no intention of allowing APR in Europe without a fight.

An opinion piece by Tatev Hovhannisyan in 2021 displayed the full panic of the pro-abortion side when faced with the reality that anyone would dare offer women a

---

[5] The website is https://povratnatabletka.si/.
[6] Brooke Myrick, "Abortion Pill Reversal Turns the World Upside Down", *Pregnancy Help News*, April 3, 2025, https://pregnancyhelpnews.com/abortion-pill-reversal-turns-the-world-upside-down.

second chance at choice. The author wrote, "'It can't be happening in Europe!' This was the first reaction of my European friends and colleagues when they heard about our team's findings—how doctors globally, backed by US religious conservatives, are providing women with an unproven and potentially dangerous treatment that claims to 'reverse' a medical abortion." The author further detailed the mental angst: "While coordinating our investigation into APR in Europe, I became sad and miserable."[7]

Unfortunately, measured, intellectually honest evaluation of the evidence supporting the safety and effectiveness of APR has been supplanted by hysteria and ideology in many countries around the world. Instead of engaging, they persecute, prosecute, and attempt to entrap.

---

[7] Tatev Hovhannisyan, "Euroviews: Europe's Regulators Must Ban 'Abortion Pill Reversal'", *Euronews*, June 18, 2021, https://www.euronews.com/2021/06/18/europe-s-regulators-must-ban-abortion-pill-reversal-view.

Part 2

8

"Three Baby Dads— That Doesn't Look Good on You"

By Sarah Hurm

I never thought I would go through with an abortion until my youngest child's father told me that it was the only option. I was a mother of three children, and I had no help from either of the fathers. My older two children's father was abusive; my third child's father had some legal/criminal issues, and I thought it was best to focus on my children and distance ourselves from him.

I was living on government assistance at the time: Section 8 housing, Medicaid, food stamps, and childcare assistance. I was working mother's hours at a doctor's office. I wanted to spend time with my children and raise them, but I also needed to work to provide for them.

In April 2018, I reconnected through social media with an old high school crush, and we hung out anytime I didn't have the kids. By May, I realized I needed to take a pregnancy test. That test was positive, but I took another just to be sure. That one was positive too. As soon as I saw those two little lines, I started crying. I just broke down right there in the bathroom. I remember falling to the ground and wondering, *How is this happening? What am I doing with my life? Why am I back in this situation?* I started to think of how everybody else would view me.

I decided that I just needed to reach out to the father. I was hoping for a supportive, level-headed response. He said we needed to be responsible adults and take care of this in a responsible way.

He meant abortion.

He told me that he was not ready for a child and that I could not take on another child. He said it was the best option for both of us.

Then I voiced my concern that I didn't think abortion would be a good option for me. I remember in seventh grade religion class when they showed us the little model of the fetus, the unborn baby. I knew it was a baby. I had also heard that sometimes abortion can be rough on a woman. But I had also heard the lie that eventually, over time, you can get over it. I think that's when that seed was planted that maybe I could have an abortion and still be okay.

Then he said, "Twenty-six years old, four kids, three baby dads—that doesn't look good on you." I believed him because those were the exact same thoughts that I had, and the fact that he voiced them out loud made them real to me.

I caved, and I called Planned Parenthood. When I called, I asked for counseling because I wasn't ready to make an appointment for an abortion. But they told me they do not offer any type of counseling. They just wanted me to either schedule the type of abortion I wanted or not schedule an appointment at all.

So I scheduled a chemical abortion. I chose the chemical abortion route because I was hoping to have a more discreet encounter with Planned Parenthood. I wanted to keep it a secret. I didn't want anybody to know what I was doing to end my pregnancy, which I had not told anybody about. On May 24, 2018, I went to Planned Parenthood in Des Moines' Southside. I went by myself. I remember walking up to the building and looking around, making sure there was nobody there praying because I knew it would make it that much harder. I also didn't want anybody to see me going in. As soon as I walked into Planned Parenthood, I met a security guard who asked what I was there for. I didn't want to tell him, so I just told him I had an appointment. He made sure I didn't have any weapons. I went up to the front desk and told them I had an appointment. They clarified and said, "You're here for an abortion, right?" I agreed, and they asked for payment.

It was $730. I had Medicaid insurance, which didn't cover it, so I paid the fee by myself—the father of the baby had promised to reimburse me for half the cost. Then they told me to just go ahead and have a seat. My appointment was at 11:00 A.M.

I remember sitting there watching the clock. Waiting was torture. I wanted to be called back as soon as possible because I did not want to think about what I was getting ready to do. I remember there was a couple sitting in front of me and another woman or two sitting alone on the other side.

It was very white and sterile, but it was grayish blue at the same time. It was like there was a filter over everything. As I was taking it all in, I was called back. It was 11:25. After the urine sample, I went into the ultrasound room. Before the door was even shut, the technician asked, "Do you want to see the screen? Do you want to know if there are multiples? Do you want to know if there's a heartbeat? Do you want pictures?"

I said yes to everything.

As soon as the ultrasound started and an image was on the screen, she turned to me and said, "You're lucky the heartbeat bill hasn't passed, because if it had, you wouldn't be able to continue." She said, "You're about five weeks, five or six days, and we have a really strong heartbeat. And if that bill was in effect, then I would have to tell you we cannot continue."

When she told me that, I remember just looking up at the ceiling, looking at the light, trying not to cry, because with a previous pregnancy, I had made a promise to God that if there was a heartbeat, I would continue with the pregnancy.

I told the ultrasound tech that I wanted to continue, but I stopped looking at the screen. All I could hear were the father's words: "Twenty-six years old, four kids, three baby dads—that doesn't look good on you." After the ultrasound, the tech handed the pictures to me in an envelope and I went to the next room. A nurse was sitting at a computer, and she asked me a bunch of health history questions. She asked me about eating disorders, cycles—all that type of stuff. And then she asked only one time (that I remember) whether this was what I wanted to do and whether the father knew I was there. I just told her that I needed to do this and that the father knew I was there— that he wanted me to come. But I never once said this is what I wanted to do or that I felt it was a good decision. I kind of danced around the question and was honest at the same time.

After I had answered all the questions, the doctor came in and the nurse turned on a camcorder on a tripod and told me I had to face the camera. The doctor was going to watch me as I took the first drug of the regimen, which I did. Then they handed me the infamous brown bag and I just walked out. I felt like I had been there forever, but in reality it was probably about two hours. Outside, it was a really sunny, hot, humid day—so different from the gray, cold place I had just been. I was immediately hit by the sun and the heat, and that's how quick and hard the despair and regret hit me. I got to my van, whose air conditioner had recently gone out, and I broke down.

I thought, *What did I just do?* It was like a switch had flipped or like I'd walked from darkness into light. I knew I was trying to kill my child, and I knew it was not the decision that I wanted to continue with.

I was crying pretty heavily at this point and was grateful that I lived nearby. When I got home, I was still crying so I decided that I would write out how I felt. And then maybe after journaling or whatever, I might feel better. I thought maybe I just needed to get my emotions out right away. So I wrote down my first journal entry to my child.

May 24, 2018

My Little One,

I am so sorry. To me, you were an alive, perfect little creation, and I wanted to hold you so much.

I know I had a choice in this, but your father didn't want to have a baby in this messy life of mine. I pray God forgives me for this because I don't know if I ever will. I pray Mary welcomes you and watches over you.

Mommy loves you so very much, and I am so sorry.

I will think of you daily and hope to one day meet you in heaven.

I am sorry, my little one.

I love you.

I will love you always.

Mama

P.S. The process is one pill today and 24 to 72 hours later another four. Baby, what if I just don't take the next four? Do you think God could help save this? Save you? I will do my best, baby. I will do what I can.

After I wrote the journal entry, I did feel a little better. I was able to realize I still had other children to care for and a life I had to live. So I picked up my three kids from daycare and school. I was hoping that picking them up would be a welcome distraction from what I had done earlier that day.

But I realized it was a lot harder not to think about what I had done that day. Looking my kids in the face was the hardest part. I could talk to them only if I was facing away from them—or they were facing away from me. I couldn't look into their perfect little faces knowing that the drug I took was trying to kill my littlest baby. And I couldn't stop the tears.

After the kids were in bed, I went online and googled a bunch of different questions: What if you don't continue a chemical abortion? Can you reverse an abortion? What happens if you don't go back to Planned Parenthood after you start a chemical abortion? Because I do remember, right before I left, they told me I had to continue. They said once I took the first drug in this regimen, there's no going back, and I needed to schedule an appointment for an ultrasound about three or four weeks later to make sure the abortion was completed. So, I was researching what would happen if I didn't.

I saw this hotline, and it looked like it was some California number. I wondered whether the number was real and whether it would be helpful to me in Iowa. Still, I told myself if I wasn't feeling better by the morning, I would call them to see what they had to say. It wouldn't hurt just to call.

The next morning, I woke up, went to the restroom, and felt like something wasn't right. I panicked. I called the hotline and heard a very sweet voice right away on the other end of the line. The nurse asked me where I was calling from. I told her Des Moines, Iowa, and she told me they actually have a provider that's just twenty minutes away. She said, "Let me call you right back. I'll see if they can get you in this morning." When she called back, she asked whether I could go that morning. I said yes. I got my youngest ready—she was about one and a half at the time—and then we went to see Dr. McKernan. When we got there, my daughter was sleeping, and I was carrying her. Katelyn, the doctor's assistant, asked, "Can I hold her?" We had to do an ultrasound. Katelyn sat holding Kalilah throughout the entire ultrasound. And Dr. McKernan looked at me during the ultrasound and told me there was a heartbeat and we could try to save my baby, but he couldn't make any promises. I told him I didn't need any promises—I just needed hope. I needed to do everything I could to try to reverse the worst decision I had ever made. At that point, we discussed abortion pill reversal, what it does, and why he wanted to make sure there was a heartbeat before we moved forward. It was the Friday right before Memorial Day weekend.

He told me about progesterone injections, and I had my first injection there in the office. He told me that I would need to do a few more throughout the weekend. And then after the long weekend, he would do a blood draw to make sure my HCG levels were increasing the way they needed to, and we would go from there. I left, and I was feeling better. I felt like I had hope again. I felt like I was doing everything I could to undo this awful decision I had made.

Later, I started to feel sick. Then on Saturday or Sunday, I met up with Katelyn and got another injection. But after that one, I did reach out to Dr. McKernan to tell him I was really sick and couldn't continue with the injections. I asked whether there was another option for treatment. He said, "Let's do the blood draw and make sure your HCG levels are increasing and it's working. And then I will call in an oral prescription for you, and you can just do the oral progesterone."

That next week I went for the blood draw, and we got the results we wanted. He called in the oral progesterone, and I started taking the progesterone pills. Then I had an ultrasound the following week to make sure the baby was growing and things were looking okay. And once we got to that ultrasound, I was definitely feeling more confident that the pregnancy was going to continue.

But then I also had to face my fears related to continuing the pregnancy. What were people going to say? But I definitely felt like I could handle facing that more than facing the regret and despair of taking my child's life. At that point, I told the father that the abortion did not work. I did not tell him I was doing the reversal. I just told him it didn't work. I was not going back for another abortion, even though he tried to convince me to go back and do it again.

I finally told him he was heartless and he needed to leave because I was not going back to Planned Parenthood. That night we had a fight; afterward, I went out to the dam at the local lake and looked into the spillway. I contemplated taking my life that evening. I didn't feel like I was a good enough mother for the three children I had, and I still had doubts that my baby would be okay. But I walked away because I heard a little voice telling me, *I am not done with you yet.*

I started to get myself ready for having another baby. I also continued to journal just because of the emotions of pregnancy. I realized I would be facing it completely alone, and keeping it from people for quite a while was hard. But I slowly started to feel joy and excitement as I thought about having another baby. And I was really relying on God, although I didn't realize it at the time. I thought he was completely gone from my life at this point, but this pregnancy was growing a healthy baby—so God had to be with me. I just didn't realize the new life in Him that was rooting in my soul.

On January 11, 2019, I gave birth to Isaiah.

Watching Isaiah grow has just been a joy. He is so full of life. He is kind, outgoing, compassionate, and intense. I call him my spitfire. He has a full smile that turns his eyes into little half-moons. He is athletic and a devoted little prayer warrior. I have realized how important and special life is. Isaiah has a lot of personality, which our family would be missing if he was not in it. And I have found new life through giving birth to Isaiah.

I am still a single parent—to four kids, with, yes, three different fathers—but it is not something that defines me in a negative way. Motherhood defines me. And motherhood is my greatest legacy and accomplishment.

The chemical abortion was my rock bottom in life, but I have been reaching mountaintop after mountaintop since. I look at all four of my children and know I do not need to listen to the world anymore, because when I followed what the world wanted me to follow—a life of pleasure, convenience, and running—I was not happy or satisfied.

Now I embrace life and all it offers. I went back to school and am a licensed and self-employed massage therapist. I got connected with my local pregnancy center volunteering in 2020–2021 and now provide chair massages for the staff there. I speak publicly about my chemical abortion reversal and published a book with my testimony and journal entries. I also share on social media and have been able to be a listening ear to others who are in the place I was not long ago.

I have seen and lived both sides of the abortion epidemic. I saw what death can do, and I now focus on spreading the joy, love, light, and hope that can be found in embracing life.

9

God Strengthens

By Emily Sarai

When I discovered that I was pregnant, I was terrified. Like most nineteen-year-olds with an unplanned pregnancy, I feared what my parents would say or do and that I was going to be a disappointment to them and others. I was afraid about my financial future, and I was certain I couldn't financially support and provide all the care a baby needed. At the time, I was a part-time student and a part-time employee. Although I earned a decent living for a person my age, it certainly was not enough to support a baby. Living at my parents' home, I was sharing an already cramped room with my older sister. I was sure my only choice was abortion.

Every day that passed before my visit to the abortion clinic, I thought of telling my parents. I kept thinking of how I could keep my baby. In fact, I had already bonded with the tiny person inside me and would have little conversations with him, and I even told my sister and best friend, Jadrien, that I was pregnant, but fear always overcame my rational thinking.

I drove to the closest Planned Parenthood clinic the Friday after I learned I was pregnant. I was surprised that a nurse saw me so quickly and took me to a room. She had me sign waiver papers releasing Planned Parenthood from responsibility if anything were to go wrong.

Then she handed me the first pill and a cup of water to wash it down. I didn't know it then, but this pill would cut off the baby's food supply and cause him to stop growing and thriving. I stared at the pill in my hand and became overwhelmed with sadness and the feeling that I was making a terrible mistake. But again, the fear I had of being pregnant overcame all other emotions, and I took the pill.

On the drive home, I was consumed with guilt and regret. I cried the whole way. Fittingly, it also poured rain the entire night. I felt like Jesus was crying for what I had done.

When I got home, I told my sister what I had done and that I wanted to fix it somehow. We started looking online and came across a website discussing a reversal process, and it had a phone number. I was filled with hope but also doubted that it was real or attainable. Once I called the number, I connected with Elizabeth Delgado; she took my information and said she would call me back in an hour or two once she found someone who could help me.

They say the sincerest prayers come from hospital rooms, deathbeds, and those in the midst of a tragedy. Well, I know that to be true because during the time I was waiting for Elizabeth to call me back, I prayed for my baby's life harder than I have ever prayed for anything before. I felt like my soul was crying and pleading with the Lord on behalf of my baby. I know God heard my prayer because Elizabeth called me back with the answer to my prayers—Patsy and Willie from the Juan Diego Center. I had an appointment to see them at 7 A.M. the next day, which would be fewer than twelve hours after I had taken the first pill.

That morning, Patsy called me and made sure I was coming; she even asked whether I needed a ride. I took her call as a sign that I was doing the right thing. Of course, I was nervous to get injected with a substance about whose validity or safety I knew nothing, but I decided to trust the solution that God had provided me.

When I got to the Juan Diego Center, Patsy reassured me that they could save my baby and that everything was going to be okay. She showed me a model of a six-week-old baby, which was the age of mine at the time, and I was able to see how real and beautiful the baby was, even when it was only six weeks old.

I think a common misconception that the abortion industry loves to promote is that babies *in utero* are only cells, not actually people. That is entirely untrue, and when I saw that model, I couldn't believe that I had almost ended my little baby's life.

I went home that day and told my parents about having started the chemical abortion and about the reversal process I was undergoing. My mom was very receptive to my decision and came with me the next day to meet Patsy and Willie. She supported me with love during my entire pregnancy and still supports me to this day.

Everything fell into place after that, and I remember hearing my son's heartbeat for the first time around Thanksgiving. In July, I gave birth to a perfectly healthy, beautiful nine-pound, eight-ounce baby named Ezekiel, which means "God strengthens", because that's what God did. He protected and strengthened my baby against the abortion pill's effects through abortion pill reversal.

I have been forever changed into a new person because of my son and what I went through to bring him into this world. He is the absolute best thing that has ever happened to me, and I am so blessed to have him as my son. God says children are a blessing and a gift from above, and I cannot agree more. Today, Ezekiel is ten years old and flourishing in every way. He is extremely smart, particularly in reading, math, and technology. Ezekiel is an amazing big brother and is talented at the piano. He is a blessing to everyone he meets, and I am forever grateful that I was able to save him and be his mama.

I hope everyone, when faced with an unplanned pregnancy, chooses life. Thankfully, if a woman makes a mistake, like I did, she can have a second chance, which is the reversal process.

10

Mimi and Her Baby Girl

By Mimi (Not Her Real Name)

At the age of twenty-five, I found myself in a complex, life-changing situation. I was unmarried and pregnant. Coming from a traditional religious family, I felt my situation would bring shame to me and my family. In my mind, having the child was simply not an option. I had accepted the dark fate that I had to terminate the pregnancy.

With a heavy heart, I swallowed the abortion pill and drove myself home to wait for the onset of uncomfortable symptoms to follow. The first set of physical responses was incredibly painful. I found myself in the fetal position on the bathroom floor. The next day I knew the second wave of pain would follow with the second pill.

I went to work, realizing it was a pathetic attempt to get back into the routine of things. I was hoping it would cloud the reality that I was slowly killing my baby growing inside me.

My sister was aware of the circumstance. I called her from my office, choked up and absolutely shattered. I asked her, "Does it hurt the baby? Like the pill, does it hurt it? Does it feel pain?" I don't know if she knew what her response would do to my mindset and ultimately my life.

She replied, "It feels something. Embryos have nerves, even this early on."

I immediately naïvely googled "reversing the abortion pill". I called the first number that appeared, and I found my guardian angel, Miss Liz. I smile as I write this because nearly nine years later, this beautiful individual is still a part of my life and my daughter's life, with photo updates and the occasional phone call. I don't think she is fully aware of what she has done for me.

Miss Liz confirmed she would be able to help me. She reassured me God had blessed me. And truly God had blessed me. Miss Liz connected me with a physician. I often think of him as well, wondering how many lives he has impacted. From him, I received the medication to reverse the process. As a result, my body was able to hold on to my beautiful baby girl.

At one point, I went to the emergency department, as the pain was too much to bear. Seeing my baby girl's little heartbeat through the ultrasound reassured me that she was a strong survivor just like her mama.

Nearly nine years later, I can't thank Miss Liz enough. I am aware every woman has a right to her own body and her own decisions, and this was mine. I am so grateful for the resources provided and the opportunity to have my baby girl in my life and forever in my heart. I can't imagine my life without her and her big brown eyes. She will never know how badly I wanted her and needed her in my life—my sweet, sweet baby girl.

11

A Second Chance

By Cynthia Michel

I was nineteen when my world turned upside down. I found out I was pregnant. My boyfriend and I had been together for about a year, and though I cared for him deeply, we were young, scared, and far from ready for the responsibilities of parenthood. I discovered the pregnancy at a Planned Parenthood clinic. Strangely, I was calm at first, resolute even. I knew I was going to have an abortion. The abortion pill seemed like the easiest, least invasive way to end it, and I convinced myself it was the right decision. A surgical abortion was out of the question, but this? It felt simpler.

When I told my boyfriend, he was relieved. He came from a Christian family and admitted he knew abortion was wrong, but he was nineteen, like me, and he could not fathom becoming a dad at that age.

My mom was devastated to learn I was pregnant. She'd had me at age eighteen and had spent years fearing I would follow in her footsteps. When I mentioned having an abortion, she agreed, reasoning it was probably for the best. Despite being a devout Catholic, she could not bear the thought of my struggling as she had. She even gave me the $400 I needed for the procedure.

I still remember the morning of the appointment like it was yesterday. My boyfriend came with me. As I sat in the clinic, nerves started creeping in. They took me back for an ultrasound, and for the first time, I hesitated. "Can I see it?" I asked the technician. She shook her head. "I'm sorry, but that's not allowed." Her response shocked me a bit.

They handed me a small plastic cup with the first pill inside and explained, "You'll take this one here and the second pill at home in twenty-four hours."

Suddenly, my calm shattered. My stomach churned; my chest tightened. I felt nauseous, dizzy, like I couldn't breathe. "Wait", I told the nurse. "I need a minute."

"Just take the pill", she insisted. "You've already paid for it."

I panicked, put the cup down, and bolted out of the room and into the parking lot, tears streaming down my face. My boyfriend followed, alarmed. "I can't do this", I sobbed. "I can't." To my surprise, he didn't argue. He simply said, "Then we'll leave. We'll figure it out."

I paced for a bit, but eventually I convinced myself I had no choice. "I already paid", I said. I went back inside, apologized for storming out, and swallowed the pill. They handed me a brown bag with the second pill and instructions, and I left feeling hollow.

The next morning, my mom told me she was going to confession. When she came back, she was crying. She said she'd told the priest everything, and he wanted to come over to talk to me. I was furious. "Absolutely not!" I snapped. "It's too late. I already took the pill."

But the priest came anyway. He was kind and compassionate. He asked me questions—about my life, my decision, my fears. Then, almost hesitantly, he said, "I know a doctor who might be able to help reverse the effects of the pill. Would you be willing to talk to him?" I dismissed him at first. It seemed impossible. But something in his demeanor softened my resistance, and I agreed to speak with the doctor.

Minutes after the priest left, I got a call from Dr. George Delgado. He explained the process of reversing the abortion pill using progesterone.

I was skeptical, so I called Planned Parenthood for clarity. They were adamant: "The baby is probably already dead. If not, it will be severely disabled. Don't listen to anyone who tells you otherwise."

I was going back and forth, calling Dr. Delgado, asking questions, and then calling Planned Parenthood to see what they said. Confused and overwhelmed, I hung up on Dr. Delgado. I told my boyfriend what the doctor had said, and we debated for what felt like hours. At one point, I even held the second pill in my hand, ready to take it. But something inside me resisted. My boyfriend finally said, "There's too much pulling us to this baby. Let's just go see."

It was the validation I needed. I called Dr. Delgado back and apologized for hanging up on him. That evening, we met him and his wife, Liz, at their office, which, ironically, was located just down the street from the abortion clinic. The ultrasound revealed something I'll never forget: My baby was still alive. The heartbeat echoed in the room, and we all cried. After seeing my baby's ultrasound, all the fears and hesitation left my mind; I never looked back. That day, I received my first progesterone injection. For the next few months, I continued the progesterone treatment until I no longer needed it.

Today, I'm grateful to Dr. Delgado and Culture of Life Family Services. They gave me a second chance I didn't think was possible. More than that, I know this was God's plan all along. He placed the right people in my path exactly when I needed them most.

Now I'm the proud mother of an incredible son, Christian. My then-boyfriend and I married in 2014, and we've built a beautiful life together, complete with two more children. Every day, I look at Christian and see not only the miracle of his life but also the grace and mercy of God.

In December 2024, I attended a Catholic high school scholarship meeting, as we were preparing for Christian's high school enrollment. I thought of Dr. Delgado, and I had tears in my eyes because it was a moment when I realized that I was on the path that God wanted for me and that everything that has happened in my life has been because of Him and because we said yes and chose life that day fourteen years ago. Christian received the scholarship, and we were overjoyed. His life is bright, full of purpose, and overflowing with opportunities.

Not long after, Christian looked at my computer that I had momentarily left unattended. On the screen was my abortion pill reversal testimony. He instantly realized that he was the reversal baby. With joy he exclaimed, "I'm a miracle baby!"

12

We Are Chosen

By Jyale Michel

I grew up most of my youth attending a Protestant Baptist church ... most Sundays. I was baptized at St. John of the Cross when I was a baby, but that was the extent of my life as a Catholic. I think having a Catholic baptism was a Mexican tradition more than anything else.

The Baptist church was a place where I was able to learn about Jesus by means of the pastor's analogies. The pastor had a great way of speaking and weaving modern-day scenarios into the teaching of the Scriptures. I would try to apply these lessons in my life but would always end up doing my own thing. I kept Jesus in my back pocket and pulled Him out in times of desperation. I would sin and look up at the sky or ceiling and say something like "Yes, God, I'm sorry" but continue with my day. It was always a struggle for me to really want a relationship with God.

I would sometimes even pray to God and ask Him to help me want Him more. The prayer was simple and something like this: "God, thank You for everything You do for me. Please help me want You more. In Jesus' name, amen."

But I always did my own thing in the end. I lived my entire youth and early adulthood trying to emulate the cultural influences that I grew up with. I was "down for the cause". I believed the way you should act was reflected in rated-R movies and music with "Parental Advisory Explicit Content" labels. After all, that was what I watched and listened to.

I was a good-hearted kid and always impressed older folks around me by being well mannered and compassionate. However, now that I look back, I can see I never really had a backbone.

When I was with people from the church, I was inspired and hungry for more. But when I was with my friends or "normal" people in my life, I would easily fall into drinking, drugs, sex, pornography ... basically, everything you hear in vulgar rap music. I was always seeking acceptance from anywhere I could get it. I literally applied what I learned from those songs to my life. That way, I would be the "cool" kid among my peers. Bad habits ended up creating a loser kid who graduated high school late because he missed nearly a third of the school year due to ditching.

But this loser kid also had charm. I was talking to a girl while in adult school to get my diploma. I didn't like who I was at the time, especially the situation I put myself in. However, that girl didn't really care about that. She was one of the first people with whom I could be honest and open. I could be myself. She just accepted me. We got closer and ended up dating.

I remember one time in my room I prayed, "God, if she's the one, please let me know. And I really pray, Lord, that she is."

Cynthia grew up as a cradle Catholic but wasn't devout. She wasn't as bad as I was, but we indulged together in a lot of sin, especially sex.

After about a year and a half of dating, I got a call from Cynthia. She was pregnant. We discussed our options and had no idea what to do. We sought free counseling at my church, and they bluntly told us to keep the baby. We reached out for advice from family members, and they all had a different answer: "Get an abortion." They were coming from a place of misguided compassion and misapplied logic.

The reasons were all the same: You're too young; you're going to ruin your lives; you can't even take care of yourselves; do it for the baby's sake. We even had a family member give us $400 to pay for the abortion. We knew they were right.

We were both in junior college and working for minimum wage about ten hours a week. So that's what we ended up doing. I pulled God out of my pocket, looked up, and said sorry. But I wasn't as much sorry to Him as I was just sorry to be in that situation.

The "treatment" we decided to go with was the abortion pill. The way it worked was that the woman would take one pill at the clinic, which was designed to kill the baby. Then twenty-four hours later, she would take a second pill to flush the baby out. They said it would be like a heavy period. It seemed simple.

I was there with Cynthia to show support. I secretly wanted the abortion, but I never said so. Instead, I told her it was her choice. But I know I was just being a coward and couldn't admit it. It couldn't be me who signed this baby's life away; I didn't want to be blamed for this. Besides, what if there were any repercussions or backlash? All that would end up falling on me. At least I could be there for Cynthia to support *her* idea, and she couldn't resent me for influencing her to make this decision.

She took the pill on a Friday at noon. We both went home and gave each other some space. We agreed that I would visit her the following day, also at noon, so I could be there for her while she took the second pill.

Well, my dad loved Saturday morning chores, so I was stuck doing yard work. It seemed like the faster I worked, the more my dad wanted to do that day. He didn't know that Cynthia was pregnant or about the plans we had just executed.

Noon passed, and I was still working. Cynthia was blowing up my phone with calls and messages, but I wasn't near my phone to answer her.

I was stressed, irritable, dirty, and tired. But I had to save face for my dad, or else it would be a whole other drama if I started giving him an attitude. So, I just kept my emotions to myself and worked as fast as I could.

It was around 1:00 P.M., and my phone was still pinging and buzzing from Cynthia's missed calls and messages. I finally picked up the phone to hear my scared girlfriend crying, thinking I had abandoned her. I ranted for a second about my dad, then reassured her that I was on my way. We were both super stressed about being late for the twenty-four-hour deadline. The nurses at Planned Parenthood were very clear about taking the second pill twenty-four hours after the first one. I headed straight for her house and finally got there at about 2:00.

When I got there, Cynthia had just gotten off the phone with a doctor. She had a lot on her mind and gave me the scoop on what was going on. She told me that her mom had gone to confession that morning and repented for giving us the money to carry out the abortion. The priest had come to Cynthia's house. He had talked to her and asked her questions about how she was feeling and why she wanted the abortion. She stuck to the rehearsed script and repeated the things that we knew and what everyone else had told us. The priest was very nice and nonjudgmental. He listened sincerely. I think this is what helped Cynthia lower her guard.

As Cynthia was telling me about her conversation with the priest, I asked her, "Well, what did the priest say?" I was expecting to hear the same stuff we heard from my church, ready to shrug it off and accept that the damage had already been done. But she told me that this priest knew a doctor who supposedly could reverse the abortion pill.

"How?" I asked. "The doctors at the clinic said once you take the first pill, there's no turning back, and if you don't take the second pill, you will have complications."

Cynthia told me that she had just gotten off the phone with the doctor right before I arrived and that she had actually hung up on him. As Cynthia and I talked, the doctor called again, but I spoke with him this time. He told me how his treatment could work. He invited us to come to his office and get a free ultrasound right then—on a Saturday night. I told him I needed to think and would call him back.

My mind was racing. I had thought this was over and the second pill was just a formality at this point. It was already two and a half hours past the twenty-four-hour deadline. The baby must be dead. Why did I need to make this decision all over again? What if the baby was alive but deformed from the first pill? I wouldn't be able to look this kid in the eye. I wouldn't be able to live with myself.

We had already had a whole week of stress and back-and-forth decision making. I was tired. I didn't want to do this anymore. I felt I was over-seeking counsel from my pastor; I was over-praying about it. This was supposed to be over with, a done deal. I just wanted to go to sleep and forget all this, but I couldn't. I had my scared girlfriend looking to me for answers that I wasn't prepared to give. I needed answers myself.

I called the doctor back and voiced my concerns. I hated the fact that we had to choose this all over again. It was supposed to be done, but the doctor still had hope.

We got off the phone again, and Cynthia and I talked to each other. We were both extremely stressed. I constantly rubbed my face and hair. There were so many pauses of silence, looking at the floor, with a question in our minds that was repeating over and over again: *What are we going to do?*

Then I felt something strong rise within me. I was a nineteen-year-old kid who was about to become a man.

In my head, I told God, *Okay, but You gotta promise me that You're going to help me. And You'll always help me provide for this baby.*

I was scared yet comforted at the same time; my fearful thoughts weren't so loud anymore. I didn't have the road map, but I knew I was about to head the right way. I knew in my heart that I would be okay, that my new family would be okay.

Then I looked at my girlfriend and said, "There's too much fight for this baby. So, this is what's going to happen."

I wasn't asking. I was confident. I was sure. There was a triumph within me. I had finally found my backbone and stood taller and firmer than I ever have in my life.

"We are going to call the doctor back and get that ultrasound. But know this, Cynthia, there *is* going to be a heartbeat, and we are going to have a baby."

We got to Dr. Delgado's office, and sure enough, there was a heartbeat. And it was strong.

Cynthia was on the table; her mom and I were next to her, and we cried as we saw sound waves on a monitor and heard a loud repetitive swishing. I wasn't surprised. I closed my eyes and looked up at God and thanked Him. I had held up my end of the deal, and He proved He was going to hold up His.

Right away the doctor put Cynthia on a treatment plan: two progesterone shots a week. Cynthia has a phobia of needles, so this was quite the penance for her.

The next eight months were a hustle. I didn't know what I was going to do, but I knew it would work out. I tried to find any work I could do while remaining in school, doing odd jobs, but it wasn't sustainable. I was barely making enough to cover gas.

I remember I had one last $20 bill to my name when I was invited to attend a Protestant church, whose pastor I didn't trust very much. I had gone there a few times before and wasn't into the loud stage music and showiness. He seemed very materialistic, talking more about money than about the gospel.

Coincidentally, the Sunday sermon was about money and tithing. It was very hard for me to buy into it, especially when I was broke. I told God that I didn't trust this pastor but that I trusted Him. With a deep breath, I took the last bit of money to my name and offered it to Christ, pleading that He would multiply it for me, reminding Him of His promise. Soon after, I got a job at Costco, with full benefits. I worked the night shift, which fit perfectly with my school schedule. Man, does He deliver.

There was also a lot of planning and talk going on about the baby during that time. A noteworthy topic was the baby's name. I didn't like the names Cynthia was throwing out, and I no longer accepted this "her body, her choice" nonsense. I was fully invested and saw this baby as much mine as it was hers. I wanted our baby to have the name Christian, which is my middle name, but she didn't like it.

Another battle we had was about baptism and the faith we would have as a family. I wasn't about to be a multifaith family. Coming from a Protestant faith, I didn't believe in infant baptism, and I would call Cynthia out for being a Catholic only because of her upbringing. I was sure I would sway her into coming to my church. I would tell her that she just wanted the baby baptized because of a cultural tradition—like it was just some juju good-luck water. But after much discussion and debate, I offered a proposition to Cynthia. I said that if we named the baby Christian, we could baptize him.

"Deal", she said. Her response had no hesitation, much quicker than I ever expected.

But I'm not someone to just do something blindly. I need to believe in it or at least have an understanding of it. So, I decided to investigate the Catholic faith. I went to my pastor and the priest who connected us to our new family doctor.

I spent several days going back and forth from St. Rose of Lima Catholic Church to New Hope Community Church in Eastlake. I asked questions about Mary, forgiveness, baptism, and other things. I learned that a Protestant baptism is similar to a Catholic confirmation. Since I knew there was a confirmation option, I was on board with baptism for my son.

I called Cynthia on the way home and told her I was totally okay with baptizing our son. And I also said, "By the way, we are Catholic now." Once again, I planted my foot firmly as I declared it.

Four years later, we got married. Before doing so, I completed the Rite of Christian Initiation for Adults program (RCIA), received my First Communion, and got confirmed at St. Rose of Lima.

Now, I won't say this is a happily-ever-after story. Marriage is very rewarding but tough. There are still several challenges that I face on a daily basis. I could ignore these challenges and even run away from them. That was definitely my strategy back in 2010. But it's the struggle that makes us holier. We are all blessed and called to be blessed. But the true fruit of the blessing comes from trusting in

God. It is through trust in Him that we are enabled to receive the blessing.

I don't deserve my son, my wife, or my other children. I did nothing to earn this. I basically just said yes after saying no a whole bunch of times.

I had been doing what I was supposed to do in order to be accepted, cool, and successful in the eyes of the culture. When I was facing the most important decision of my life, people who legitimately cared about me and wanted the best for me were advising me based on their perspectives and experiences. However, as logical as their arguments may have seemed, they were actually steering me away from God, the real truth.

I challenge you men reading this to look within yourselves. Are you living in truth? I thought I was, but I really wasn't.

As His beloved, we need to be aware of how we human beings, who are full of fear, anxiety, and insecurity, are in need of His blessings. I was blessed by that doctor who said yes to seeing us on a Saturday night. I was blessed by my mother-in-law who humbly said yes and went to repent. I was blessed by the priest and pastor who counseled me. And although I didn't realize it at the time, I was blessed to be baptized and marked as a child of God.

And it's not over. My son is a fifteen-year-old blessing. This blessing is going to want a car soon. This blessing lives on, and he is one of the first cases to prove that the abortion pill can be reversed. My hope is that this testimony helps people like my then-girlfriend and me so that they can have hope and choose life.

It may be tough. It may be uncomfortable. But it definitely will be worth it. Tough times don't last, but tough people do. And when you are walking with God, you are indestructible.

Fast-forward to 2025. I am married to the same courageous woman. Last year we celebrated our tenth wedding anniversary. We have three beautiful and healthy kids who go to Catholic school, and we are regular participants at a Traditional Latin Mass parish in San Diego. As a family, we grow in love through the Church, walking with God, and basking in His mercy.

13

From Abortion to Reversal to Public Speaking

By Rebekah Hagan

In early 2013, my life took an unexpected turn when I found out I was expecting my second child. At the time, I was eighteen years old, a college freshman, newly single, and already raising an eleven-month-old baby boy. The news of another pregnancy felt like a crushing blow. I had fought so hard to prove everyone wrong, and here I was proving them right—that I never did learn my lesson, that I was reckless and broken. I had left an abusive relationship and was determined to create a better life for my son and myself. But now I felt like I was on the verge of losing everything I had worked for.

The fear was overwhelming. I imagined my future slipping away—my education, my independence, my dreams. Worse, I knew that my network of support would likely disappear. My family and friends had struggled to accept my first unplanned pregnancy and had just come around, and I couldn't imagine putting them through it again. I felt completely alone, drowning in shame and uncertainty.

Desperate for a way out, I convinced myself that abortion was the only responsible and compassionate choice. I had grown up in church, but now my faith felt distant—completely overshadowed by panic and fear. A chemical abortion seemed like the least painful option, both physically and emotionally. It was marketed as safe, private, and natural. I wouldn't have to undergo surgery or explain my decision to anyone. I could take a few pills and pretend this had never happened.

I walked into the abortion clinic when I was just over seven weeks pregnant. A nurse explained the process in a clinical, quick, and detached manner. She emphasized that once I took the first pill, there was no turning back—the pregnancy would end. I nodded in agreement and signed some forms. Then she handed me a brown paper bag filled with the second round of medication, misoprostol, and told me to take it at home the following day. The only instruction was to call if I experienced blood clots larger than a lemon.

I swallowed the first pill, mifepristone, feeling as if it were the only way out of this awful ordeal. But as I walked to my car, regret hit me. My hands shook as I gripped the steering wheel, my heart racing. *What did I just do?* The weight of my decision hit me—I had started something I desperately wanted to undo. Had I just made the worst mistake of my life? Was there any way to fix it?

Embarrassed and ashamed, I knew I could not walk back into the abortion clinic for help. Instead, I turned to my phone and began frantically searching for a way to undo the abortion pill process. After what felt like forever, I found the Abortion Pill Reversal (APR) website, which had launched just a few months before, and called the hotline. Nurse Debbie answered, and later in the process, Nurse Liz spoke with me. I'll never forget them. They met me in my mess, offering reassurance and a plan. While I cried, Debbie explained that mifepristone blocks progesterone, the hormone needed to sustain pregnancy, and that reversal aimed to treat my body with progesterone to counteract mifepristone's effects. While there were no guarantees, the chance to save my baby was worth the effort.

They worked quickly, making call after call until they found a doctor in Northern California, a kind, gentle godsend of a provider close to where I lived, who was willing to help when others said all hope was lost. Less than twenty-four hours after taking the first pill, I sat in his office, starting the progesterone regimen. I stayed on the treatment for several weeks, hoping and praying it would be enough. I wanted to believe everything would be okay, but the fear never truly left me, not for another thirty-two weeks or so.

In October of that year, my second baby—a little boy—was born and is one of the first documented abortion pill reversal success stories. He was, and still is, perfectly healthy.

Today, our lives look nothing like they did all those years ago—thank God! I graduated college on time, with two toddlers in tow, watching their mama walk the stage. My younger son is growing into an incredible young man—curious, kind, and full of life. He's heading into his teenage years, which comes with new challenges but also so much joy. He's always at the top of his class, has a sharp sense of humor, collects comic books, runs his own small business, and is musically gifted, like his older brother. Most importantly, he has a heart of gold and is known for his compassion toward others.

Looking at my younger son today, I can't help but think about how close I came to missing out on him. Without the help of abortion pill reversal, I wouldn't have the privilege of knowing and raising one of the most incredible human beings I've ever met.

The good news does not stop there. I'm now married, and my husband and I have been blessed with two more children, making us a family of six. Our home is filled with laughter, noise, and all the beautiful chaos that comes with raising four kids. Beyond our family life, we have dedicated ourselves to helping women facing unplanned pregnancies. My journey led me to a calling I never could have imagined—I now speak full-time, sharing my story across the country, encouraging women, guiding students, advocating for pregnancy help organizations, and equipping churches to walk alongside those in crisis.

I'm deeply grateful for abortion pill reversal and the brave providers who offer it. They give women like me a real chance at choice—one that goes beyond what feels like an irreversible decision. APR was a lifeline when everything seemed hopeless. It didn't just reverse my abortion; it saved my baby and my future. It gave me the space to rethink my path, make better choices, accept grace for the poor ones I'd made, and start fresh. Every day, when I look at my son and see the redemption that has unfolded in our family, I thank God for this second chance—one I never expected but will always be thankful for.

14

Abortion of Twins: "Am I Making the Right Decision or Not?"

By Terri Corado

It all started in July 2018 when I sat up in bed one morning and became nauseous almost immediately. I instantly knew I was pregnant since I had experienced the same feeling twice before. Quickly, I rushed to the store and purchased a pregnancy test. It confirmed what I had already suspected.

My first thought was not of excitement but rather fear, stress, worry, and not knowing how I would tend to another baby when I already had two. I was already a single mom, already divorced. We lived with my grandparents, and I was working as a bartender/server, barely getting by. I was in no position mentally, physically, or financially to bring another innocent baby into this world.

I called the man I was dating at the time, who is now my husband, to break the news that I was pregnant. He was speechless. He assured me everything would be okay, but I didn't feel the same. Our relationship was anything but perfect. I called him one day expressing my feelings about the entire situation, explaining that I had done some research and believed abortion was the best option for me. He disagreed and wanted to continue the pregnancy. My family was not supportive of my having another child and pushed me to have an abortion. I knew deep down it wasn't the right thing to do, but at that time and in that dark place, it seemed like the only option I had.

I made an appointment at my nearest Planned Parenthood, feeling scared and sick about the decision I was about to make. I was depressed, lonely, and sad. After walking into the building, I checked in. They called me into the back after a short time in the waiting room. I didn't go to the normal exam rooms, though; I went into a part of the building that was cold, much colder than the office as a whole. It was a feeling of sin, evil, and death, and it was weighing heavily on me. I knew I was making the wrong choice, but with my family pushing me, my already complicated situation with the baby's dad, financial strain, and the fact that I was a young adult, I tried to ignore my intuition and gut feeling and decided to continue with the plan.

The nurse walked in and asked whether I wanted an ultrasound. I said yes, despite knowing that it would make this difficult decision even more difficult. We continued with the ultrasound and the nurse asked, "Do you want to know the number of fetuses?"

I said yes. She said, "There are two." Shock, disbelief, and absolute heartbreak weighed on me heavily. I started shaking, but I told myself to continue with the plan.

I went into this all-white room, with nothing in it besides a table, chair, medicine cabinet hanging on the wall, and a laptop computer on the table. I sat in the chair and the nurse walked in and turned the computer on. The doctor connected for the appointment virtually and asked me a few questions. Then the nurse handed me the abortion pill. I was told that I would take the first one in the office and that it would slowly cut off all supply of life from me to the babies. The second pill I would pick up from the pharmacy, and that would assist in the passing of the babies. The doctor and nurse were cold. No emotion whatsoever.

I swallowed the pill and walked out. I got into my car and cried; I couldn't talk; I could barely stand. I was disappointed in myself, disgusted, and numb, and I had thoughts of harming myself so I wouldn't have to live with the decision I had just made. I called my boyfriend and told him that I didn't want to live anymore, that I had made the most awful decision. I was so ashamed of myself. I don't remember much of that conversation other than his just supporting me, trying to calm me down, and offering to help me find a solution. He said there had to be a reversal—something that could stop the abortion. I just kept repeating, "What have I done?"

Later that same day, I searched online for something to reverse the first pill. I came across the Abortion Pill Reversal website and knew I had found what I needed. I called the hotline number and spoke to someone on the other end of the line. I remember crying and explaining to her what I had done. The lady I spoke with was patient, kind, and reassuring; she told me that she would help get me in contact with someone locally who could help me. I remember feeling a weight lifting off my shoulders almost immediately. A little later, I was put into contact with a local women's center, made an appointment, and went in feeling lost but hopeful.

I was connected with Dr. Dewey, my angel. She prayed over me, guided me, loved me, and supported me; I will be forever in her debt. She was light in the darkest time of my life. Dr. Dewey explained the reversal pill and how it works and told me that she would try her best to reverse the first pill. I was prescribed progesterone to take at home until I reached a stage in my pregnancy where the babies were out of danger. Every single appointment I had with Dr. Dewey and her staff was so calming. When my pregnancy was no longer in danger, I had my last appointment with Dr. Dewey. I remember how she prayed yet again over me, my family, my pregnancy, and my kiddos; then she gave me the biggest hug. I cried and scheduled an appointment with an obstetrician to continue prenatal treatment. Dr. Dewey not only saved my babies; she also saved me.

My babies now are six years old, and they are thriving every day because of this reversal, because of people like Dr. Dewey and her team who invest their time into women who are broken like I was. I couldn't be more thankful for this reversal and for everyone along my and my kids' journey who prayed over us, listened, and guided us to where we are now.

15

From Russia

By Natasha (Not Her Real Name)

Translated by Dr. Alexey Fokin

Before this pregnancy, my husband and I already had three children, and a fourth child was not included in our plans. It was a shock for me and for him.

On the advice of my friend, I called a clinic and was scheduled right away for a chemical abortion. All this happened very rapidly, so I did not even have time to weigh everything.

When night fell on the day I took the first pill, I was left alone with my thoughts and began to think that quite a long time had passed since taking the first pill—and that surely it had already begun to work. It was at that moment, when I lay so relaxed in my warm bed, that I realized that the pill was killing my child. Or maybe my child had already been killed.

I felt unbearably sorry for my baby. I understood, at that moment, that an innocent child was dying. This baby came to be through the fault of my husband and me. It was not her fault that my life was difficult. It hurt a lot. I sobbed, went to the internet, and without any hope began to google whether it is possible to reverse a chemical abortion.

I called gynecologists, and they all told me in no uncertain terms that it was impossible to stop anything. Then I found a site called peredumala.ru (which means "changed my mind"). It talked about the techniques used to reverse the effects of the abortion pill. And they had a link to their social network. I reviewed a lot of information in it and then wrote directly to the coordinator of this group, Anna. I told her my situation. She helped me throughout my pregnancy.

I started taking progesterone almost a day after taking the first pill. I ran straight to the pharmacy, then wrote to Anna that I had taken what she had prescribed. She said that I was doing everything right.

After seeing that the baby was alive and growing, I felt great joy that I managed to at least reach this stage. That I had done everything I could to prevent a negative outcome. I was relieved that she was alive, that the pill did not affect her, that she continued to grow.

Despite all my fears, my baby was born absolutely healthy. Over the years, I have never regretted that I decided to give birth to her, that I gave myself the opportunity to have a child again. I love this child very much. I am grateful to her that she has made me a hundred times happier than I was before.

16

I Felt Like a Single Parent in a Two-Parent Household

By Mary Doe (Not Her Real Name)

I was a mother of two when I found out I was pregnant. My younger child had just turned one, and my relationship with her father was falling apart. I felt like a single parent in a two-parent household, and I knew all responsibility would fall on me if I had another baby.

I went behind the father's back and made an appointment to get an abortion. The day came; I had a heavy feeling in my chest while waiting to receive the first abortion pill. The doctor knew I felt unsure but gave me that first pill anyway, which I took in front of him.

I went back home and could not stop crying about what I did. I kept crying to those I trusted most, and I was not sure about taking that second pill. They told me it would be difficult to raise three children on my own and that I should go through with the abortion.

The next day at 10:00 A.M., twenty-four hours had passed, and my alarm was going off to take the final pill, but I couldn't. I called Planned Parenthood and told them I did not want to go through with it. They advised me there was nothing I could do but take the second pill. I called my OB, and I was turned away.

I was feeling hopeless, but I wanted to save my baby. I spent over three hours making phone calls and googling how to reverse an abortion pill.

I found the APR hotline, and Debby, the nurse at Birth Choice, was the first person I spoke to. I'll always remember that moment and the hope I felt that I could possibly save my baby. I was prescribed progesterone immediately to reverse the effects of the abortion pill.

The next day I had an ultrasound to check on the baby. The moment I heard the heartbeat, I broke into tears, relieved that everything was okay. It was unbelievable seeing my baby being so active at only eight weeks.

I continued to take progesterone and went in for weekly ultrasound visits with Birth Choice until I was thirteen weeks. Birth Choice has become family since then, providing materials and resources for me and my kids.

My healthy baby boy, Joseph (not his real name), was born on May 5, 2024, and he was the chunkiest baby I have had yet. He had full cheeks and a cute little nose. He was perfect to me.

I cannot imagine what my heart would have carried for the rest of my life if I did not fight for my little one's life. Introducing my miracle baby to my Birth Choice family was a special moment in my life. I will forever appreciate their love and dedication to me and my children.

I once read something that said, "You will always regret not having that child, but you will never regret having another child." And I could not agree more.

17

A Grandfather's Perspective

By Rich

As far as I remember, my daughter disappeared for a couple of days when she found out she was pregnant almost ten years ago. When she returned home, my wife discovered that she had been to a Planned Parenthood earlier that day. My daughter told her she had taken RU-486 (mifepristone). Apparently, her boyfriend at the time had talked her into going there, and I think he was in the room at Planned Parenthood to make sure she took the abortion pill.

She said that she really didn't want to abort her baby and told us there might be a way to reverse it. Then she handed us the other medication, which was supposed to be used on day two. My daughter's sister was also present. None of us were familiar with any of this.

I went to my computer and googled "RU-486", and everything popped up concerning this, including abortion pill reversal with a contact number. We called the number, and Liz answered the phone.

After we shared with her what had happened and she explained what our options were, she had a local physician in their network contact us. The doctor talked to my daughter, arranged an appointment, and prescribed the progesterone needed to reverse the effects of mifepristone.

We had to drive seventeen miles to the pharmacy that was open all night. At that time, I knew that Liz was our family's guardian angel, including for our granddaughter who wasn't born yet. She helped set us up with the physician for further treatment a day later.

My daughter was monitored from that day until the child was born. Later in the pregnancy, my daughter had a complication and Liz helped us through that. My granddaughter and many other babies would not be here if it weren't for Liz and George Delgado and the center in California they are associated with. Someone has to be an advocate for the unborn.

18

The Very First Known Reversal

By Matthew Harrison, MD

Thursday afternoons at our clinic were usually when we started to wind things down for the week. It was late in the morning, and I received a call from the front desk at Northgate Family Medicine. There was someone on the line from the local crisis pregnancy center, and she wanted to speak with me.

Dr. Danny Holland had started the practice two years earlier as a natural-family-planning-only clinic, meaning that he did not prescribe birth control and did not refer for abortion, sterilization, or in vitro fertilization, all in accord with the teachings of the Catholic Church. At the same time, he had built a reputation as a keen diagnostician and hardworking doctor who took a personal interest in his patients, often caring for multiple generations.

Delivering babies as a family medicine doctor was becoming harder to manage, but it was a blessing to be able to take care of the mother and the baby in the hospital as well as in the clinic. We had good relationships with the pregnancy centers around Charlotte, North Carolina, because we had been offering free prenatal care and delivery services for abortion-vulnerable women for quite some time.

When I got on the line, the pregnancy care center worker said that she had a young lady who had come to the office and had taken the abortion pill but then changed her mind. The desperate mom wanted to know what she could do to save her baby. Could anything be done? At that time, chemical abortions were so new that I had no idea what I could do. But the best thing is always to meet face-to-face and offer any help you can, so I asked her to send the young woman right over.

Amber (not her real name) was my first appointment after lunch. She was nineteen years old and distraught. Amber said that she had been in an intimate relationship with her boyfriend, who had always promised that if she ever got pregnant, he would support her and her baby. She was reluctant to be intimate with him because she came from a Christian family, but she loved him and thought that they would spend the rest of their lives together. This was a scenario very familiar to me, as I have seen many young ladies looking to build relationships but finding themselves compromising their standards in a culture that so heavily endorses physical intimacy over spiritual and ethical intimacy.

When she did become pregnant, he backpedaled immediately and told her to get an abortion. The boyfriend threatened, "If you don't get an abortion, your parents will not understand and will kick you out of the house! You will have to quit school and will never fulfill your dreams."

He said that he would not support her and her baby. Instead, he gave her $265 to go to the abortion clinic and have it "taken care of".

These are fear tactics that we hear very commonly, and as a result, vulnerable women take desperate measures. Sure, I've met women who choose abortion lightly, solely for convenience, but the vast majority are caring young women who see abortion as their last and only choice. Many are driven to self-hate, and their decisions, made under extreme duress, are akin only to something as serious and final as suicide, in some way killing a part of themselves in search of relief for the pain and fear they are experiencing. Many women are shamed into getting abortions, and their shame keeps them from healing ministries to get past this loss in their lives.

Amber went to the abortion center and reluctantly kept the appointment. The abortion center staff estimated her pregnancy to be just over seven weeks, but they did not let her hear the heartbeat or see the baby on ultrasound.

Seeing the ultrasound images and hearing the heartbeat are critical for a woman to make an informed decision about her pregnancy. Studies consistently show that when a woman hears a heartbeat and sees her developing baby, she is much more likely to choose life and find a way to support that child. Laws that require women to see the preborn baby or hear the heartbeat are not there to punish but rather to guarantee that all the information about the pregnancy is available.

Amber did not get this chance to see her baby or hear its beating heart. They handed her a little white pill, mifepristone (RU-486), the abortion pill. She was instructed to take it right there, and they would not let her leave before taking it. After she took the pill, they gave her the misoprostol to take forty-eight hours later to induce contractions. Her encounter was confirmed by our clinic when we received her records.

Amber immediately felt regret. She left the abortion center hoping she could throw up or somehow get rid of the drug but could not. Immediately, she went home and could not bear the thought of what she had done. Amber knew it was wrong, and her regret mounted.

Twenty-four hours went by, and she was getting desperate. Her Christian formation helped her realize that what she had done was wrong.

She initially called the abortion center; a staff member told her, "There is nothing that can be done. You better take the second pill, and you better come back in a week to get checked. If you don't finish this and the baby survives, it will be physically deformed or developmentally delayed." So much for the compassion of the abortion industry. We still hear these lies coming from abortion providers, completely unfounded and unscientific medical advice.

Thankfully, Amber finally went to her mother and told her what had happened. To her relief, her mother was supportive and loving. She said, "Let's see what we can do to get help."

She wanted to do anything she could to help her daughter and her grandchild. So they went to her local crisis pregnancy center, Cabarrus Women's Center. Once there, they explained the situation and then were sent to my office.

I was pretty amazed by the story. I had never heard anything like this. I was familiar with the abortion pill, that it had been FDA approved in the year 2000 and was gaining widespread use. We were now in the summer of 2006, and it was being used in about 20 percent of abortions.

But I was also perplexed. I had no idea what to do in this situation. This is not the type of thing they teach in medical school. But I've always known not to give up and not to make snap decisions in emergency, life-or-death situations. Amber had not yet started to bleed or cramp.

I asked her to excuse me as I went to my office and thought about it. I literally prayed to God for guidance. I pulled out the *Physicians' Desk Reference* and reviewed mifepristone's mechanism of action. I read that it was a powerful progesterone blocker that was initially created as an adjunct cancer treatment for hormone-dependent tumors that can't be resected. Mifepristone is a progesterone antagonist; among other actions, it attaches to the progesterone receptors of the placenta without activating them, thus leading to a separation of the placenta from the lining of the uterus. A tight adherence is required to supply nutrition and oxygen to the developing embryo and, later, fetus.

So I was sitting in my office, poring through the *Physicians' Desk Reference* to figure out how mifepristone works and how I could counteract it. And then it hit me. The abortion pill works by blocking the progesterone receptor in the lining of the uterus. Because of my background in biology, specifically protein-receptor mechanics, I understood that mifepristone could be outcompeted by an abundance of progesterone that could reactivate the progesterone receptors. If progesterone was the key to unlock and activate the receptor, mifepristone was like a bad key that would not only fit in the lock without activating it but also block good keys from entering the lock. If we supplied enough good keys into the patient's system, we could override the bad keys blocking the progesterone receptors.

We had progesterone in our office because we were using it in fertility care treatments for women who had naturally low progesterone levels. My practice partner, Dr. Holland, was a certified natural family planning medical consultant trained in NaProTECHNOLOGY through the Saint Paul VI Institute in Nebraska, led by Dr. Thomas Hilgers. Progesterone has been safely used in pregnancy for over fifty years, mainly as a supplement for women with luteal phase defects, which cause low progesterone levels and increase the risk of early miscarriage.

This novel antidote for a mifepristone abortion had never been used before, as far as I knew. I was reassured knowing that progesterone was safe in pregnancy, especially the bioidentical type that we used at near physiological levels.

I took the idea to Amber, and she was ready to do whatever it took to save her baby. I explained to her the risks of the abortion completing and of the baby remaining in her and possibly causing infection. I told her we would need to very closely follow her to make sure they were both doing well.

She consented to the treatment, saying that she would try anything to save her baby's life. We gave her an injection of progesterone and hoped for the best.

The next day she started to bleed, and we asked her to go to the emergency room for an ultrasound, as ours was not available that day. The ultrasound showed the formation of a blood pocket (called a subchorionic hemorrhage) on her placenta, which was starting to separate from her uterus. She was, however, able to see her baby's heartbeat for the first time. Later, she told me simply seeing her baby's heartbeat would have made the treatments worth it. The emergency room doctor told her to go home and hope for the best.

By the fourth day after initiation of the reversal treatment, Amber had stopped bleeding, and she came by our office. We were able to confirm a heartbeat, and we continued progesterone replacement. The progesterone had outcompeted the mifepristone, and the placenta had healed!

With a half-life of eighteen hours, the mifepristone was now completely metabolized out of her system. The rest of her pregnancy was unremarkable. She continued progesterone replacement therapy until about twenty-eight weeks.

When Amber was forty weeks, she gave birth to a beautiful baby girl, Katie (not her real name). She had no birth defects, and her placenta was normal, as verified by the pathologist. Today, Katie is a healthy, bright seventeen-year-old girl.

So now what? Was it a fluke? There wasn't a good way to test this. I was a family medicine doctor, so this was a tiny part of my very busy practice, and I really didn't know where to turn with this information. But every month I looked forward to those well-child checks when Katie would come to the clinic, and I got to witness her grow into a lovely young lady. Amber was so heroic and humble and remains so to this day. She doesn't really want a spotlight and remains happy with what she wanted all along, a sweet life with her sweet daughter.

And the threats that her boyfriend made? They amounted to nothing. Amber solidified her relationship with her parents, who supported her throughout the pregnancy, and she was able to complete her education while raising her daughter. She is now working in the health-care field herself, saving the lives of NICU babies. Amber is a living example of how moms can carry their pregnancies to term and fulfill their dreams as well. Abortion is not the only answer; there are people who can help.

19

Above the Clouds: My Perspective as a Hotline Nurse and Nurse Practitioner

By Kathryn R. Grauerholz, MSN, NP

It was the spring of 2012 and an intense season of conversion in my life when I attended a prayer breakfast for Catholic women. I had never been to one of those events before, and I was ambivalent about attending since the speaker, a nurse, was also a pro-life advocate at a pregnancy care clinic. My apprehension arose from the personal injury that I had suffered from an act of violence in my teen years that had caused a lot of darkness in my life. I was just starting to recover from post-traumatic symptoms I had endured for many years. The incident did not include pregnancy or abortion, but for some reason the topic of abortion was a trigger for my anguish. I avoided anything that involved the topic of abortion, pro-life or not. That day, I had decided to attend because I was going through a very healing and spiritually fruitful time in my life, and the friends who were supporting me during that time were sharing a table together. It was out of a sense of gratitude to my new friends and the Lord that I wanted to attend.

The speaker, Debbie, shared her tremendous spiritual conversion story and described her work as a nurse in a clinic that helped pregnant women who were abortion vulnerable. She described her experiences as a provider of early obstetric sonography and some of the life-affirming conversations she had with women. I had a hard time listening because it was triggering symptoms in me; at the same time, I felt my heart on fire within me. I had the burning conviction that the work she was describing was what I was being called to do. Nonetheless, I didn't want to listen, and I didn't want to participate in something that had been so unpalatable for me. The prayer breakfast ended with praise and worship. I felt compelled to approach the woman who spoke to my heart, but I resisted that day.

I continued on a trajectory of healing and spiritual growth, but I became more hardened and resistant to participating in pro-life work. During that time, I had also begun to meet regularly with a priest who provided spiritual direction. Several months after the prayer breakfast, I was planning to hike up a local mountain with a friend. She canceled last minute, and I decided to climb it anyway. I started the ascent up the mountain that was shrouded in foggy clouds. When I made it to the top, I found myself above the clouds. In the clarity of the moment, I enjoyed the surrounding beauty and spent a good amount of time in contemplation and prayer. I descended the mountain with a galvanized conviction that I was meant to participate in the pro-life work that Debbie described at the prayer breakfast.

At the urging of my spiritual director, I quickly got to work by praying peacefully outside abortion facilities. Then I learned how to assist women as a sidewalk counselor, which I did for a couple of hours every week for several years. So much good was accomplished by these simple efforts. I was profoundly impacted by the gratitude of some of the people who wanted to discuss life-affirming alternatives to abortion. It was as if the shadowy gloom that had hung over me for years was dissipating and being replaced by a new clarity and purpose.

About a year later, at another prayer breakfast, I saw Debbie, and I told her how profoundly her testimonial had affected me. She was thrilled to learn of my interest and agreed to help me. We continued to run into each other at various events, and she offered me advice that helped me along.

Not long after Debbie's initial and moving presentation, Dr. George Delgado, the physician she worked with, formulated an abortion pill reversal protocol and started the hotline program. Over a few years, Debbie had become an integral part of that work and was an assistant in his research. She introduced me to this work, and I was trained as an APR hotline nurse who answered questions and phone calls from women who were interested in reversing their chemical abortions after taking the first drug in the two-step process. In that time span, I also met Dr. Delgado, and he casually told me that I could come and work at his family medicine practice/pregnancy care clinic anytime. I applied for open positions and was turned down three times over several years. I was told it was because I was credentialed as an adult nurse practitioner, and they were looking to hire family nurse practitioners.

In the meantime, I continued to work as an APR hotline nurse for several years, while simultaneously working as a full-time nurse practitioner in hospice and then as a nurse educator of programs that focused on pregnancy-loss grief care. Over a decade after having the initial conviction that I was to do the work that Debbie described at the prayer breakfast, I started as a nurse practitioner at Dr. Delgado's practice and currently perform ultrasounds and care for patients who are seeking APR or are vulnerable to abortion.

New Beginning

My first shift working as an APR hotline nurse fell on the feast day of Saint Maria Goretti, an eleven-year-old Italian martyr and model of chastity. Immediately after I logged in, numerous calls poured in. I had to call Debbie, the shift manager, who provided me with assistance and training throughout the day. Even with the two of us working together, we were overwhelmed by the volume of calls. The first caller resided in an area where only one physician was listed as available, and then we found out that she was on a leave of absence from her medical practice. We started calling Catholic churches in the area and searched for leads to locate another physician. Finally, after several hours, we were able to locate a physician who was very willing to partner with the hotline and provide APR in that region. She continued to provide progesterone to patients in need for years after that encounter.

That day, another caller urgently wanted help but was caught up in continuing her workday and other responsibilities. I urged her to head over to the available obstetrician as soon as possible and informed her how important timely initiation of the treatment was. She didn't start the progesterone until the next day. When I called her on the third day, she was crying and reported that she was bleeding and had stopped taking the progesterone. I inquired about the bleeding and urged her to seek continued advice from the provider prior to discontinuing the progesterone. Then between sobs she told me that she lost the baby in the shower. She was very disturbed by encountering the physical form of the baby's body. She didn't know how to handle the remains or her anguish. I was shaken by her grief and trauma. This terrible outcome and her anguished response left me feeling totally unprepared and despondent. I did my best. I expressed my heartfelt sorrow for her loss and offered her resources for grief after pregnancy loss.

On that same day, another caller, Dawn (not her real name), told me she was desperate to get started on the progesterone to reverse her chemical abortion. After I had gathered her information and described the process and procedure, she was quick to respond and willing to drive an hour to get to the appointment with a provider of the APR regimen. She had initiated the chemical abortion because she was not in a stable relationship, had concerns about her ability to parent, and wondered whether she had the financial means to raise a child.

After taking the first pill in the chemical abortion process, she immediately regretted her decision. She expressed that all her concerns seemed irrelevant when she realized she would end the life of her child and never get the chance to hold her baby. After taking the mifepristone, Dawn instantly acknowledged that she was already a mother. At once she was shaken by the realization that she would lose her baby forever. She wanted to start over as her baby's mother. She wanted a second chance. When I spoke with her after she had seen the health-care provider, she tearfully told me that her baby was still alive and that she saw the heartbeat on the ultrasound. I journeyed with her through the abortion pill reversal.

For the first week, I called her daily, then weekly through the first trimester, and then monthly. Of all the encounters that I had the first day as an APR hotline nurse, her baby was the first to be born.

When I began as an APR hotline nurse, the shifts were twenty-four hours and there was no additional support staff to filter the calls prior to my receiving them. I often received several calls a day from women or men seeking to obtain abortion pills. They typically hung up or even cursed at me when they found out that I was offering life-affirming alternatives to abortions and not mail-order chemical abortion pills, which were not approved by the FDA at that time. I remember how long that first shift of calls was and how it continued through a long night. I probably had only an hour or two of uninterrupted sleep. The dreams I had during those short rest periods brought me to the foot of the Cross in the Lord's Passion. The dreams and all that happened during that first shift only reaffirmed my conviction that this work was indeed what the Lord was calling me to do.

In Flight

It was about midday when I got the call from Salina (not her real name). I was on the other line with a physician for another client when she called. After the other call ended, I attempted to call her back several times unsuccessfully. It always distressed me to know that someone who needed help wasn't getting it in a timely manner.

Finally, she answered, and she said she was in the middle of filling her car with gas. She briefly told me she would call me back soon before hanging up on me. When she finally called back, she told me she was at the airport and almost ready to board an airplane. She was taking her three kids to another state to visit her brother. At that time, she was nearly nine weeks pregnant and had taken mifepristone thirty hours prior. Her demeanor fluctuated between desperation and casualness, which was strangely conflicting. On one hand, she urgently wanted to reverse the abortion; on the other, it seemed that she didn't want to face the reality that she had initiated the abortion of her baby, as she coolly continued with her vacation plans. Salina shared that she had already had three other chemical abortions in the past, but she didn't want to go through the emotional trauma of having another abortion. The conversation was cut short as she boarded the plane with her young children, whom I could hear in the background. I was trying to impress how important it was to start the progesterone as soon as possible when the phone suddenly disconnected.

Three hours later I received a text from her that she could talk. I tried calling her unsuccessfully; a little later, I reached her. She said it wasn't a good time because she was just leaving to take her kids to the pool. A couple of hours later she called back and said the battery of her phone wasn't working well; the call might be cut short. She said she wasn't going to be able to return home to start the reversal process and wanted to initiate reversal where she was. She also said she didn't have the money to pay for a physician visit. She wanted the prescription called in to the local pharmacy. I proceeded to describe the APR process and stressed why it was necessary to be evaluated by a physician and have follow-up ultrasonography. She agreed but said she had no way of paying for it. Meanwhile, it was weighing on my mind that the clock was continuously ticking, and her baby's life was on the line.

Then, God sent an angel: A physician was willing to see Salina and treat her with progesterone injections that she had for obstetric emergencies. I called Salina with the good news, but she said she was at the local theme park with her kids. She thought she might be able to go later and reasoned that her brother was giving her children a once-in-a-lifetime opportunity. I couldn't believe what I was hearing, and my mind was continuously cognizant that time was slipping away.

Much later, when I checked in with her, she had already seen the physician. I was thrilled as she told me the details and thanked me for all my help. She was elated to have seen the baby and heard the heartbeat for the first time, as she hadn't been allowed to view the ultrasound at the abortion facility. She said she was a little sore in the upper buttock area where she received the injection but was completely relieved and hopeful that her baby would live. The next day, she returned to the physician and received another injection before returning to her home state.

Because of her traveling, I had to start over again and search for an APR physician who could continue to monitor the progress of the abortion reversal and provide ongoing pregnancy care. I found another provider, and Salina was able to start oral progesterone for the remainder of the first trimester. The initial conversation with this physician went really well, but I experienced ongoing difficulty arranging her care at his office. The office staff was refusing to schedule follow-up appointments because of insurance-related conflicts.

I continued to check on her monthly, and occasionally she responded affirmatively. In the second trimester Salina said she had gone to the emergency department for cramping in her back. She was thrilled to let me know the baby looked great per the ultrasound she'd had and all was going well. She was also convinced her baby was a boy. As far as I could tell from our conversations, she never received any other prenatal care, even though I offered her several options. She always said she had insurance but couldn't afford the copays. I was relieved when Salina announced with joy and gratitude the arrival of her healthy baby boy.

Hope

I worked the APR hotline on Sundays because I had another full-time job. I was told that the volume of calls on

Sundays was typically less than other days of the week. It was Super Bowl Sunday, and I had mentally prepared for a quiet day of work on the APR hotline. On the contrary, I was inundated with calls throughout the day.

Evangelina (not her real name) called very early. I noticed immediately that her voice carried both desperation and hope. She told me how glad she was to find a method to reverse abortion. She was sure that God was guiding her call. She confided that she thought she was having a boy and that she believed wholeheartedly that the Lord would see her through the APR process and her son would survive. She had visualized his future, and suddenly she could feel her son moving and kicking (which is not common at that gestational age), letting her know that he wanted to live. Her enthusiasm and total confidence made me increasingly nervous. She had taken mifepristone two days earlier at the abortion facility and had taken the second drug, misoprostol, at home. We prayed together. Evangelina was staunchly resolved and eager to start progesterone and override the chemical abortion. I informed her that the research to date was on mifepristone reversal, not the reversal of mifepristone and misoprostol.

I immediately started calling around her area, which unfortunately was not a location with many life-affirming providers or pregnancy help centers. My efforts were further thwarted by the fact that it was Super Bowl Sunday. Finally, after much searching, I found a provider who was willing to meet Evangelina at the provider's office. The physician wanted to do an ultrasound first since Evangelina had taken both mifepristone and misoprostol.

When I let Evangelina know about the APR provider I had arranged for her to meet, she said she wanted to see a provider in her HMO group that would take her insurance. I quickly went to work to locate another provider, and it was nothing short of a miracle that I found one recently retired from her HMO network. He was not in the office and required that an ultrasound be done prior to administering progesterone. He informed me that the only option available was for her to go to an HMO-affiliated emergency department (ED) for care. Evangelina preferred to go to the ED instead of going to the out-of-network provider, so she headed that direction. Meanwhile, time was quickly passing and I feared that her baby wouldn't make it. Still, she was sure all would be well.

A couple of hours later, I checked in with her about her progress. She had waited for over an hour to be seen, but the radiology staff refused to provide her the ultrasound since Evangelina had brought her two young children with her. She was told that she would have to return without her children to have the ultrasound performed in the radiology department. This was a crushing blow to our hopes of getting the progesterone started promptly. I suggested she change her plans and see the out-of-network physician I had originally suggested. But Evangelina still insisted on getting care compatible with her insurance network. It took her some time to find a babysitter, and then she had to wait again for hours in the ED for another opportunity to get an ultrasound. It took the whole day.

It was evening when she called and asked me what to do when the doctor came to discuss the results of the ultrasound. I was starting to get ready for bed when I was called by the attending physician. I provided him with the progesterone protocol. Ultimately, he prescribed the progesterone as I had instructed. It took a couple of hours for Evangelina to get the prescription because she had to retrieve her children from the babysitter and experienced delays at the pharmacy. We were both elated when she obtained the progesterone and took the first dose. She was on cloud nine after seeing her baby move, hearing the heartbeat, and knowing that saving his life was indeed possible. She was praising the Lord, and we prayed together again. I started to feel a little bit reassured.

The next day when I checked in with her, she was thrilled to report that all seemed well. She denied any bleeding or cramping. She still felt pregnant, and some of the nausea had even returned. She still believed she could feel the baby moving and trusted all would work out because the Lord had shown her son's future to her. She was gushing with gratitude.

The following day, I attempted to reach her several times, but nothing. Radio silence. I was worried. The next day, I called again, but nothing. On the third day after starting the progesterone, Evangelina answered the phone and was sobbing when she informed me that she had started bleeding heavily and ended up going to the hospital. No viability was detected on the ultrasound. She lost the baby. She was crushed and so was I. Evangelina allowed me to pray with her and accepted my condolences and pregnancy-loss resources.

I have to admit, this was the most difficult disappointment I had experienced as an APR hotline nurse. I felt so bad. I was unable to come to terms with this devastating loss.

Then, a couple of months later, out of the blue, I received a text message that said, "Thank you for giving me hope." I didn't recognize the number and initially thought perhaps it was a wrong number or spam, but then I recalled the tragedy we had shared. My eyes welled up with tears. *What?* She had lost the baby and our hopes were crushed. After all that effort, we had lost. Perplexed, I told her I was grateful to have had the opportunity to help her and that I was keeping her in prayer.

Her response reminded me of the value of this difficult work (even when reversals are unsuccessful) and the long-term, healing impact of caring grief support. I cherish being a witness to the beauty of hope that can be found amid the ashes of grief and despair.

Lamentations

Inez (not her real name) called me at the beginning of my shift. She was tearful and frantic to reverse her abortion. Her boyfriend, Max (not his real name), was supportive of her decision to proceed with the abortion reversal process. He had not known about the pregnancy prior to the initiation of the chemical abortion and really wanted his child.

I was astonished by the ease with which I was able to contact the local physician and get the prescription ordered at the pharmacy. Within two hours, Inez had taken the first dose of the progesterone. The APR was initiated only twenty-six hours after taking the mifepristone the previous day. The following day she enthusiastically sent me a video of the ultrasound performed at the doctor's office showing her living baby. She was gushing with gratitude.

I was sent monthly reports and photo journaling of her progress. Her messages were always filled with thanksgiving for her developing child. After her son's birth, monthly updates and photos continued for the following year. She sent me Halloween costume photos and Christmas photos of her baby boy enjoying the seasons. I just couldn't get over how the easiest case provided the most enthusiastic outpouring of gratitude.

After the one-year-old photos and first-birthday tributes, I didn't hear from Inez again until three and a half years later. I received a text message that she had questions for me and needed me to call her. I wasn't working for the APR hotline anymore, but I recognized her number since she had texted and called me so frequently. I shuddered as I tried to imagine what happened. Was there something I overlooked or a late side effect of the reversal process?

When I called, Inez reported that her son was wonderful, and she loved being his mother. She was treasuring her child, but she was also struggling daily with guilt that was affecting her mental health. She explained that every day when she looked at her son with admiration, she also experienced invading thoughts that reminded her that she had tried to have an abortion. She lamented that the grip of shame and guilt was tearing her apart. Every day she was experiencing anguish that brought her to tears.

Inez had sought care from therapists, which hadn't really been helpful. Her situation was unique, and they were unsure how to help her. The invasive thoughts were affecting her relationships and her job.

Inez confided that she had sought an abortion because her employer had threatened to replace her if she was pregnant. At that time, her appearance was an important condition for her position. Inez was struggling financially at the time but never thought in her wildest dreams that she would consider an abortion. In a moment of weakness, she was desperate and afraid of being unemployed and pregnant.

Now, after understanding the importance of her child's life and parenting him, Inez was considering litigation against her former employer for threatening her and nearly ending the life of her child. She wanted to know more about the mental health ramifications of pregnancy termination and the mental health challenges experienced by those who had successfully completed a chemical abortion reversal through APR. I didn't have answers to all her questions, but I referred her back to the administrators who were now managing the hotline. I consoled Inez and told her that I believed her son would want to receive his mother's love unhindered by the shadow of guilt and shame. I also suggested she seek out spiritual healing support since she had already indicated that she belonged to a Christian community.

This was not an isolated scenario. APR providers and nurses have shared that parents with children born after an abortion attempt and successful APR, though overwhelmingly grateful to have their children, continue to grapple with guilt, loss of wholesomeness, or alteration in their relationships with others, requiring both emotional and spiritual healing.

Fruition

Years had passed since I started as an APR hotline nurse. As I mentioned earlier, I am now employed as a nurse practitioner by the organization that started the APR protocol and hotline. As part of my new role, I was trained to provide early, limited obstetric ultrasounds for pregnant patients and to evaluate patients and prescribe the progesterone APR protocol.

This time it was a Friday evening; I had just arrived home ready to unwind and start the weekend. I received a phone message and text from Dr. Delgado that a young patient was requesting a call about the APR protocol. Dr. Delgado was about to board an airplane and couldn't attend to it. I was excited to have the opportunity to help. I also received a call from the client advocate who had done the initial triage.

The patient, Tamara (not her real name), had just confessed to her parents and her boyfriend that she had started a chemical abortion by taking mifepristone. They were upset, didn't want to lose the baby, and were willing to support her through a pregnancy. She regretted not disclosing her fears and pregnancy to them before starting the abortion.

When I called, she listened only for a few minutes, answered a couple of the questions I had, and then handed the phone to her mother, who continued the conversation with me. I was able to explain the process to Tamara's mother, who was grateful. I arranged to meet with them before regular office hours on Monday morning for an ultrasound and early pregnancy care. Then I called the pharmacy, expecting to spend a long time on hold since it was late on a Friday. To my surprise, the pharmacist was prompt in taking the progesterone prescription and said that her physician was one of our providers. She expressed how much she loved having such a great primary care physician. I hadn't given her any details about why the prescription had been prescribed, but the pharmacist was enthusiastic about the early pregnancy support that is provided by our practice. I was elated to have such great receptivity and ease in this encounter.

On Sunday afternoon, I was surprised when I received a call from the client advocate, who relayed the message that Tamara hadn't made up her mind to start APR until now. She had gone to urgent care compatible with her insurance plan and had the ultrasound, which confirmed the viability of her child. I was deeply concerned that she waited so long. I got word that she finally decided to take the progesterone on Sunday and would see me the next day.

Tamara was young and pretty with a slight build. Her eyes were a little misty because she was anxious about being there. Her boyfriend and mother were there to support her. Tamara's mom did most of the talking. I was so grateful to have the ability to help them and perform the follow-up ultrasound to evaluate the effectiveness of the abortion pill reversal process. When the ultrasound image of the developing baby became visible on the screen, the young parents were so amazed by the extent of the baby's development. It was thrilling to see the baby's movements, limbs, and heartbeat. I also pointed out and explained the reassuring appearance of maternal blood flow and thickened uterine lining. Additionally, Tamara was surprised and pleased to learn about all the support that was available for her as a teen mother. She could finish the year of high school without having to continue at her current school as a pregnant mom among her classmates. Her boyfriend was motivated to complete his high school curriculum before the baby's birth and start a job to support Tamara and their baby.

I saw Tamara and her boyfriend a couple more times as she continued the progesterone until the end of the first trimester. The ultrasounds were helpful for their growth and transformation as parents. The pregnancy support persons from our organization threw her a baby shower with all the pink decorations and gifts for the baby girl she was expecting. They were amazed by the gift of a child shortly after. I am delighted and blessed to report that her safe delivery also brought to fruition my becoming an APR provider.

20

My APR Journey as a Wife and a Nurse

By Elizabeth M. Delgado, RN

As the wife of the founder of the original APR protocol and hotline, I was fortunate to experience the evolution of this life-saving program from the front row. I would not believe the successes, challenges, and triumphs of the past fifteen years had I not witnessed them with my very own eyes. Early on, I took an active role as an APR hotline nurse and walked with those women in need.

The Early Days

In 2008, when George got his first APR call, I remember asking him, "Well, do you think it can be reversed? Can you help this woman?" His response was "It's possible, knowing how mifepristone works and its relationship to progesterone."

Years before, George had completed training in NaProTECHNOLOGY, and this helped him navigate the first case. The training was intense; upon completion of his classes, I recall him saying, "It felt like I was back in medical school." Due to this expertise, he was confident that the effects of mifepristone could be reversed by flooding the system with progesterone, and, fortunately, in this case they were.

Two years later, George's first case in San Diego came via a priest. The priest had read about the possibility of reversing mifepristone and knew of George's prior involvement. He put the young woman in contact with George. The initial call took place on a Saturday morning, and there were back-and-forth calls throughout the day between the woman and George, as well as George and the priest. Each time George got off the phone, he asked me to pray. We prayed together and individually. We had plans to eat with our daughter and our future son-in-law. They understood the gravity of the situation and waited patiently as we pushed back our meeting time. All of us persevered in prayer.

Finally, very much to my surprise, the couple agreed to meet with George at the office for an ultrasound; I accompanied him, as the nurse. Upon arrival, I remember the woman's body language, especially her crossed arms and downward gaze. George talked to them for a while and then the ultrasound was completed. They were able to see and hear the baby's heartbeat. George invited them to record the sound of their baby's beating heart, and the dad did so with his phone.

The mood after the ultrasound changed. I sensed that the tension had diminished and was replaced with a feeling of peace. After she gave her consent, I gave the first shot of progesterone to the mom, and on departure we hugged each other. It had been a long day full of uncertainty, but it ended with hope. We met our daughter and her boyfriend for dinner in Old Town that evening and gave thanks to God for these beautiful couples in our lives.

Later, George said to me, "I think I need to start a hotline for women who want to reverse the abortion pill. There must be others who want to reverse." *Wow*, I thought.

That's what leaders do; they see a need and fill it. His forward thinking led to the inception of the APR hotline in May 2012. Calls were fielded initially by an employee of Culture of Life Family Services (COLFS), Vita La Fond; it was soon discovered that a nurse would be better suited due to the medical nature of the calls. The first APR hotline nurse was another employee of COLFS—my dear friend and pro-life warrior par excellence, Debbie Bradel, RN. George had asked whether I was interested, and I told him I needed some time to think about it. It did not take long, and I joined the hotline in December 2012. Calls were minimal at the beginning; this gave us time to recruit doctors, midwives, and other practitioners to join our provider list. We needed them throughout the country so that women could quickly start the reversal treatment.

I received my bachelor of science in nursing (BSN) many years ago. Our BSN program included a certificate in public health nursing. The last semester of classes focused on how best to care for individuals in the community who may not have access to health-care services. I did not think I would ever need the public health training, but what I gleaned from those classes and the related field assignments helped me connect with my APR clients. I met them where they were, listened to their concerns, focused on their strengths, and encouraged them as we journeyed together.

I found these women in a variety of situations: single, married, divorced, and between relationships. Additionally, I discovered multiple reasons for them to seek an abortion: too young, too old, school commitments, job security, financial troubles, relationship concerns, and living situations. I was there to listen, provide encouragement, assist with problem-solving, and, most of all, convey that I cared about them. One young student told me she wanted to travel to

Europe. I told her Italy is not going anywhere. She responded, "You're right," and laughed at the thought. At times, the prospect of motherhood was overwhelming for the clients, and I would say, "You have time; the baby is not coming tomorrow."

With so many pressures these women faced, I often thought of a wise psychologist who told my husband and me when we were new parents, "Be where your butt is." That pretty much sums it up. Take a deep breath and take that first step. I would say, "You would be surprised at what you can do if you set your mind to it. Believe in yourself. I believe in you."

One thing that struck me was the women who were adamant about getting an abortion. They would say things like "I knew this is what I wanted to do. I was 100 percent sure!" Then after taking the first pill, it hit them, and they regretted it. They were so surprised they reacted that way. For these women, it took an action to get their actual response; an action causes a reaction. There were also women who were hesitant before taking the abortion pill and knew, immediately after ingesting it, they wanted to turn back the clock. Thankfully, because of APR, these women were given a second chance; we were ready to help.

At the onset, getting help for these women posed some challenges. We needed to find a provider in their area willing to see them, provide an ultrasound, and prescribe progesterone. Fortunately, progesterone has been used in pregnancy for over fifty years, and it's been proven to be safe and effective. One of its primary uses is to help sustain a pregnancy in women who have suffered a previous miscarriage and have low levels. Many providers knew this and did not hesitate to help with APR; others needed more proof.

When a provider could not be found, the hotline nurses had to be resourceful. We contacted local pro-life organizations to find health-care professionals who could possibly help. On weekends and after hours, I asked the clients whether they wanted to go to the emergency department (ED) of their local hospital. If they were willing, I called ahead and asked to speak to the ED doctor or charge nurse and explained the situation. The majority of the time, they would provide an ultrasound but were not always willing to prescribe the progesterone. I advocated for these women to the best of my ability. The APR team worked tirelessly to increase the number of providers. George published a peer-reviewed article in the *Annals of Pharmacotherapy* in December 2012 to document the first cases of mifepristone reversal. This publication helped tremendously in our recruitment of practitioners. Meanwhile, women traveled long distances, sometimes up to two hours, to see a provider. It amazed me to see the great lengths these women would go to start the treatment to save their babies.

Auggie's Peeps

In late 2013, I had the opportunity to fly to San Antonio, Texas, to see our first grandchild's ultrasound. I realized that I was scheduled for the APR hotline but decided to go and take calls too. At that point, there were only three hotline nurses taking the twenty-four-hour shifts, and I didn't feel comfortable asking one of the other two nurses to cover for me. Besides, the number of calls we received was still minimal. When the ultrasound day arrived, it happened to be my busiest call day thus far! Prior to the appointment, I juggled calls and spent time with my pregnant daughter. When we got to the doctor's office for the ultrasound, I stepped outside the waiting room to take a call from a woman in

Tennessee who was pregnant with twins. Initially, I was worried that I would not be able to get a provider due to it being a twin pregnancy. I completed the intake with the client and called Dr. Paul Gray. He reassured me that this was good news because twins produce much more progesterone and reversal was probable. He agreed to help the woman. I arranged everything with her, and just as I hung up, my son-in-law waved to me to come see my grandchild on ultrasound. God's timing is perfect.

Later that evening, when my daughter and I were ready to watch one of our favorite movies, *Emma*, I got a call from a young woman named Emily from the San Jose, California, area who wanted to reverse her chemical abortion. With limited computer access, I called my husband and asked whether he knew of anyone in that particular area of Northern California. He enthusiastically said, "Call Willie Lapus, the director of the Juan Diego Center. He contacted me not too long ago and said they were ready to help with APR." Word of APR was spreading throughout the pro-life communities in 2013! I called Willie and experienced firsthand how a pregnancy resource center could handle an APR case quickly and efficiently. Patsy, a volunteer from the center, called Emily and asked whether she needed a ride to the appointment. Emily went to the center the next morning. The doctor saw her and administered the progesterone. Willie and Patsy were present and provided Emily with the support and resources she needed.

A few months later, George and I had the pleasure of meeting Emily and her family while on a trip to Northern California. We also toured the Juan Diego Center and met Willie and Patsy in person, spending many hours collaborating with them on how best they could help grow the APR program. They set up a meeting with a local ob-gyn and another pregnancy resource center. Both the doctor and center joined the APR Network.

Because of people like Willie and Patsy, the APR program expanded. Willie passed away a few years ago; before he died, he said that his involvement with APR was one of the greatest achievements of his life. I am grateful to him and Patsy for arranging the meeting with Emily since our encounters with APR clients are solely over the phone. I was also fortunate to hear Emily's testimony at the Juan Diego Center's annual dinner. The powerful impact of her heartfelt words of gratitude, relief, and joy she expressed regarding APR could not be emphasized enough. I have kept in touch with Emily over the years and have enjoyed watching her sweet son, Ezekiel, grow. He and our grandson Augustine (Auggie) are the same age. After Emily's case, when I would have to end a phone conversation with my daughter due to an incoming APR call, she would say, "Go save Auggie's peeps, Mom." We are a family.

Trials and Triumphs

The first two weeks after a woman starts the progesterone for reversal are met with trepidation, yet hope. Most of the time, our clients experienced some bleeding. We prepared them for this, telling them that if they did experience bleeding, it didn't necessarily mean they had lost the baby. Follow-up ultrasounds that revealed a viable pregnancy brought so much joy and relief for these women. I shared in their joy, while giving thanks to God for using me as His instrument. With each woman's permission, we prayed to God for His guidance and loving care.

Not all the women who called the hotline experienced a successful reversal. I told them, "No matter the outcome, you were courageous in making the call to the hotline, and you tried." I offered resources for pregnancy loss to help them heal physically, spiritually, and mentally. These resources included the international organization Rachel's Vineyard and, locally, Rachel's Hope in San Diego County. Both offer retreats for women who have experienced an abortion. Some women started the reversal process, then changed their minds again and continued with the chemical abortion for a number of reasons. Pressure from family members, friends, or the father of the baby would often cause them to reconsider.

Not surprisingly, some women would contact the abortion clinic where they took the initial pill. Often, the women were given erroneous information. "No, it can't be reversed." "You signed the paperwork; you need to finish what you started." "There will be birth defects."

One of the saddest stories was from a woman who told me she had called the clinic to tell a staff member she didn't want to take the second set of pills and wondered whether she could continue her pregnancy. The staff person said that it was cruel of her to consider such a thing and explained that it was like shooting your dog and then watching it slowly die.

Women seeking to reverse their chemical abortion often rode a roller coaster of emotions. The initial call inquiring about APR was often accompanied by the concern, "If my baby survives, will it have birth defects because of what I've done?" In these situations, it was important to correct misinformation they had received. It helped us greatly when the American College of Obstetricians and Gynecologists (ACOG) came out with its statement on mifepristone and teratogenicity stating that "no evidence exists to date" that mifepristone, RU-486, causes birth defects.[1]

---

[1] "Practice Bulletin No. 143: Medical Management of First-Trimester Abortion", *Obstetrics & Gynecology* 123, no. 3 (2014): 676–92, https://doi.org/10.1097/01.AOG.0000444454.67279.7d.

Some cases were challenging, and there was one case in particular that was difficult. The young woman started progesterone for reversal and then experienced some heavy bleeding for which she received medical treatment. I received a call from the client's father who told me he didn't think the baby would make it. The heart rate was low. Yet, with determination, the mom persisted in her treatments and later gave birth to a healthy baby girl. I tell this story because the client's father has kept in touch with me through the years by sending greeting cards for holidays, occasional updates, and texts of thanksgiving for helping his family. He cherishes his granddaughter and can't imagine life without her.

Often we do not hear from our clients after our initial contact because once they get connected with a provider and pregnancy resource center, our work is complete. It is a blessing for me to get a photo along with an update from a former client. On the day of our son's wedding five years ago, we had just left the church and were headed to the reception when I got a text from a woman expressing her gratitude for my help in saving her son. I was feeling emotional because I had just witnessed my son say "I do" to his wife, and I imagined this woman having the same experience with her son in the future. I said a prayer of thanks to our Lord for this sweet text. I will always feel connected to these families whether I hear from them or not.

I continued to take calls over the years, and our fledgling APR program at COLFS in San Diego grew to the point that it needed to be taken over by a larger organization. In April 2018, Heartbeat International took the reins. I remember the month and year well because "our baby" grew up: APR '18. I stayed with the hotline until early 2023, assisting women all over the United States and many foreign countries. Women who call the hotline can now be assured they will be connected with a local provider within an hour's drive.

Over 7,000 babies have been born because of APR, and this all began with a woman who started an abortion and then changed her mind. She sought help; no one coerced or pressured her. Considering this, I don't understand the firestorm that ensued because of APR—the attacks and criticism of the use of progesterone to counteract the effects of mifepristone. As the saying goes, "It's just progesterone." They called the new science junk science, denying and ignoring that every new discovery starts somewhere. Saying that women never change their minds is laughable. Even if only one woman decided to pursue reversal, all our efforts would be worth it: a place on the family tree for the precious survivor. APR came to be because of a need, because of people willing to take a chance. I am so very thankful for the opportunity to have helped these courageous women and their precious little ones.

All of us in APR said yes to the call.

> Wait for the LORD;
> > be strong, and let your heart take courage;
> > yes, wait for the LORD! (Psalm 27:14)

21

The First APR Hotline Nurse

By Debbie Bradel, RN

After praying the Stations of the Cross at my local parish in the spring of 2011, my family and I walked over to enjoy the fish fry in the hall. As we lined up at the buffet table, I heard, "Hi, Debbie! Guess what? Did you know Dr. Delgado is looking for a nurse to coordinate patient care at Culture of Life Family Services? With your passion for the preborn, I bet he would hire you!"

I replied, "Hi, Molly! No, I hadn't heard! I am still working part-time for the County of San Diego as a public health nurse, but I am looking around for something else because they are eliminating part-time positions, and since my kids are still young, I don't want to work full-time."

"You should check it out."

"Thanks, Molly! I will! Let's eat some fish!"

By Easter 2011, I was the pregnancy care coordinator at Culture of Life Family Services, the only Catholic family medical practice in San Diego with a ministry department focused on providing free medical care to abortion-minded and uninsured women. Primarily, I took referral calls from local pregnancy help centers to schedule their clients at our clinic for urgent pregnancy medical conditions such as early pregnancy bleeding. Additionally, we saw pregnant women considering abortion. We would provide emotional and medical support, including ultrasounds, to allow them to see the new life growing inside them. We never promoted an abortion decision because of our faith-based practice, and we never coerced them into choosing life.

The part-time position I held at the County of San Diego prior to taking on the position at COLFS was as a public health nurse in the Maternal Infant Health Department. I visited young, underserved families in their homes to teach health and safety with a goal of preventing child abuse and promoting healthy pregnancies and birth outcomes.

One year later, in May 2012, Dr. Delgado asked me whether I wanted to help him start the abortion pill reversal program. I was thoroughly delighted to accept the rare opportunity to work alongside another champion for life.

If there had already been an APR program in place when I began my nursing career in 1976, it would have been my number one choice of nursing work because I passionately believe abortion hurts women. I have always wanted to prevent abortion with all my heart. So, I was grateful to be asked to help start such an impactful program.

The first APR program tasks were to build a directory of providers, start a dedicated 24/7 hotline, create a website, and write policies and procedures. Volunteers and paid staff members scoured NaProTECHNOLOGY and pro-life physician directories to recruit doctors from all over the world to sign up with us to assist pregnant women who had taken mifepristone (RU-486) but had regretted their decisions and wanted to keep their babies. There were websites with directories of physicians listed as natural family planning medical consultants and holistic women's health providers. There were lists on websites for the Catholic Medical Association, American Association of Pro-Life Obstetricians and Gynecologists, Christian Medical & Dental

Associations, and My Catholic Doctor. There were Catholic parishes with doctors who advertised in their bulletins and mom's group ministries whose leaders happily told us who their favorite doctors were who did not provide abortions or contraceptive prescriptions. Each morning our team would be excited to see who could sign up the most doctors from these lists. Sometimes providers said "No thank you" because initially we did not have a study published. The providers who signed up typically were familiar with prescribing progesterone for early miscarriage prevention.

To be listed in the APR physician directory didn't require any payment nor was there any financial benefit; it just meant the provider would take the call to speak with the woman seeking help. Once the provider obtained consent from the woman to receive reversal treatment, the doctor could call in a prescription and set up an appointment for an ultrasound in the clinic as soon as possible.

Calls came in slowly at first, so being on call by myself 24/7 didn't become too demanding until late fall 2012. That's when Dr. Delgado suggested his wife, Liz, join me in taking calls. Looking back, putting several nurses on call from day one would have been smart, but by being the only one on call for six months, I immersed myself in the program and fell in love with the opportunity to listen with understanding and compassion to the men and women who called.

One time I went into my bedroom closet to take a call at 1 A.M. from a New York woman who had undergone a surgical abortion and thought it could be reversed. In between her sobs, I tried to console her, knowing there was obviously no medical treatment available for her request. Many women had immediate regret, but most calls came at night when emotions tend to rise. The hardest part was trying to beat the clock to get a provider to pick up my call fast enough before the woman started to doubt we could help her. The most common fear was that if the baby was saved, he might have birth defects. However, the abortion pill does not directly attack the developing embryo; instead, it destabilizes the endometrial lining so that the placenta slowly becomes detached.

Another serious challenge was gathering data to build our evidence base since we were not seeing most of the women in our own clinic. It is likely that some babies were saved that we didn't know about because some women would stop answering our calls. But once we had documented hundreds of cases, we had ample evidence that the APR success rate was very good.

From 2012 to 2019, I took hundreds of patient calls and trained nearly one hundred professionals to become APR nurses. I learned way more than I did in any other nursing position about prenatal care and counseling. Later in this time period, I was granted the extreme blessing of being trained to provide early pregnancy ultrasound to confirm viability, dating, and location of the embryo for abortion-minded women as well as APR clients who came into our clinic.

I have heard many heart-wrenching stories from women who considered abortion, and I can see why people think it's compassionate to offer abortion services as an option to women in crisis pregnancies. Little do they realize that abortion is the last thing a woman needs in a tough situation, as it is not a healthy solution.

It has been extremely rewarding to maintain contact with my APR nursing colleagues and many of the women who called, both those whose reversals were successful and those whose reversals were unsuccessful. I have remained a mentor for one lady who was making a living as an escort when she took the abortion pill in 2016. Unfortunately, she was in the 30 percent cohort of unsuccessful reversals. Over the years, talking weekly, I have seen her go from aimless, angry, and anxious to positive, prayerful, and purposeful. She suffers from a chronic illness that is too debilitating to allow her to work; an older son contributes to the rent, and she is reimbursed by a government program to provide care for her ailing mother. She, like many of the women whose cases were unsuccessful, always expresses joy that she tried.

A majority of the women who called the hotline and spoke to me stated they were religious. Their moral compass pointed them back to their spiritual reality when they went in a completely opposite direction by choosing chemical abortion. One of my most memorable cases fits in this category. She was a nursing student and vocalist at her church but got tangled up with a man who enticed her with his money and influence. Once their relationship went to the physical level, she realized he didn't really love her, but it was too late. A baby was on the way. Her decision to abort their baby was based on her paralyzing fear and anxiety of having to marry a selfish man and not being able to start her career as a nurse. Her decision to abort completely darkened her mind and soul, and the cloud wasn't lifted until she took the first pill and realized that she had completely departed from her Christian beliefs. She desperately wanted the chance to go back and change her course. Soon, she found me on the APR hotline, where she received the reassurance that progesterone treatments would give her the chance she was looking for to turn back the hands of the clock and undo the decision she had made in a state of panic.

Later, she told me my support and that of the provider I found for her gave her peace knowing that God loved her unconditionally. His mercy helped her trust Him, regardless of the outcome. Her deep dive away from God followed by His mercifully pulling her out of the depths of her despair had a huge, lasting impact. Even though her baby did not survive the abortion pill, she survived a wrangle with the devil, returned to her faith, and is now expecting her fifth child, with a man of faith who loves her beyond her expectations. She not only finished her undergraduate nursing degree but also went on to get her family nurse practitioner degree and has a manageable work-life balance. Most importantly, she is now as close to God as she could be. She told me God brings good out of our mistakes if we invite Him to help us.

One of my favorite things about being an APR nurse is receiving pictures of the babies who were saved and are growing up all over the United States. Not a month goes by that I don't hear from a handful of parents who kept my number. They are so grateful for the second chance at life they received that they just have to share their gratitude and joy. They all say they think the progesterone made their child super smart. Of course, there is no proof of that, but as their virtual grandma, I lightheartedly agree and share their joy.

As APR continues to be available, accepted, and offered to women who, like all of us, deserve a second chance when we make a mistake, I continue to cherish the opportunity I was given to assist women in saving their babies' lives and doing what I could to lessen the regret for women whose reversals were unsuccessful.

22

Dr. Delgado's First APR Case

By Terri and Tim Palmquist

Erin once thought she would never consider abortion. In 2007, this young mother in Texas did not realize that the heartbreaking crisis she was about to experience would lead her to do the unthinkable.

Her deepest desire had been to be loved and wanted by her husband, but when he abused and abandoned her, she felt broken and unwanted. Erin had recently found comfort by trusting in the love of Jesus Christ, but she still felt the need for a man to fill the void in her life. Soon she met another man who made her feel like she was loved and wanted again. Although deep down she knew her relationship with him was wrong (and that he wanted her only for sexual gratification), she had no other Christians in her life to help guide her. Within a few months, she was pregnant—and soon she was abandoned again.

Erin's pain was exacerbated by the realization that she would now be a single mother—and that terrified her. As the only child of a single mother (with whom she had a very difficult relationship), she desperately hoped to avoid repeating the same negative cycle for her beloved baby.

Having no job and no means of support, Erin felt very alone. Her financial problems had made it necessary for her to live with her mother, even though their relationship was still difficult. After a couple of weeks of agonizing in secret over her pregnancy, she finally broke the news to her mother. To Erin's relief, her mother responded with kindness and compassion, but then she offered Erin $400 to abort the baby. Erin was shocked, but her mother tried to comfort her by minimizing the impact of abortion, saying, "You're not the first, and you won't be the last", insisting that Erin's life would be better if she sacrificed this child.

Erin knew that her mother meant well. Although she didn't want to abort her baby, Erin also didn't want to reject her mother's generous offer, feeling that she had no other option. "The enemy kept telling me that I couldn't provide for this child", Erin recalled. Having no job and no other means of support, Erin still wanted to believe that God was greater than the devil and that she could somehow find a way to save her baby. But her mother's offer seemed to crush that hope.

After a failed attempt to find help through a local organization, Erin felt that she had no other option than to make an abortion appointment. Reluctantly, on a Wednesday morning in May 2008, Erin went to Planned Parenthood, where she was administered a mifepristone (RU-486) pill to kill the ten-week-old baby in her womb. She didn't realize that, at the time, FDA regulations prohibited the use of mifepristone after seven weeks of pregnancy and that Planned Parenthood was intentionally violating FDA standards (though eight years later the FDA revised the guidelines for mifepristone to allow its use at up to ten weeks of pregnancy). After Erin swallowed the pill, Planned Parenthood sent her home with another drug, misoprostol, telling her to insert it vaginally in twelve hours to complete the process of removing the (presumably dead or dying) baby from her uterus.

With each hour that passed, Erin kept thinking that her baby might still be alive. As the time approached for her to insert the misoprostol, she couldn't escape the overwhelming conviction that she wanted to try to save her baby. But now she didn't even know if that would be possible. She started panicking, fearing that she was too late, but she had to at least try.

Erin called Planned Parenthood, pleading for a way to save her baby, explaining that she had changed her mind. But instead of accepting Erin's choice and providing the appropriate care, Planned Parenthood violated their own motto (which states "care, no matter what"), choosing instead to scare Erin, claiming that if she tried to save her baby, she would likely suffer a serious hemorrhage and could even have a heart attack and die.

But Planned Parenthood's switch from care to scare tactics didn't stop Erin. She was still determined to try to stop the abortion process before it was too late. "I prayed to God, and I said, 'Lord, I don't know what to do'", Erin recalled.

During the final hours of that day, Erin began searching on the internet for a way to save her baby. Several times she found phone numbers for pro-life help organizations, but every time she called, she had the opportunity only to leave a voicemail message. Her crisis was far too urgent for her to wait for someone to call her back, so she didn't leave any messages. Instead, she kept searching.

Eventually she came across our website for LifeSavers Ministries, a small, local pro-life group that we established in 1984 in Bakersfield, California—almost a thousand miles away. The motto displayed across the top of this website was "saving babies, one heart at a time". That was exactly what Erin was looking for: someone who could help save her baby. *If they really save babies, maybe they can save mine*, Erin thought. Seeing my name, Terri Palmquist, along with the toll-free phone number for LifeSavers, Erin hoped that I would answer the phone even though it was so late at night.

I had long been accustomed to taking urgent phone calls in the middle of the night from desperate women. Years earlier, we had installed a phone on the front porch of the LifeHouse pregnancy center, and some of our most desperate, life-saving calls came from that porch phone because back then many people did not have cell phones. I and other LifeSavers volunteers also often gave my phone number to abortion-bound women at the Family Planning Associates (FPA) abortion center located across the street from the LifeHouse.

When Erin called late that night, I was busy getting my children ready for bed, but I knew that I needed to immediately stop what I was doing to focus on Erin's crisis. Our children were accustomed to situations like this, knowing that when I had an abortion phone call, they had to be quiet and patient no matter what was happening.

Never before had a woman asked me how to save her baby from the abortion pill. When Erin first explained her situation, I actually didn't know what could be done. Nevertheless, I told Erin not to worry, having faith that I would somehow find a way to help her. While Erin poured out her heart to me, my husband, Tim, looked in our literature library for a pamphlet titled *Survivor*, written by Debra Braun from Pro-Life Action Ministries, which tells the story of a woman who decided to try to save her baby by not using misoprostol even though she had already taken mifepristone. That baby, named Kameryn, was born healthy, but Kameryn's mother had an extremely difficult and painful pregnancy because she hadn't taken anything to counteract the effects of mifepristone.

DR. DELGADO'S FIRST APR CASE

Without a moment's hesitation, Erin insisted that she was willing to endure months of pain and sickness to try to save her baby. Erin said that even though she knew the outcome might not be good, she had to try. "I wanted to do the right thing, even though I had already done the wrong thing", Erin confessed.

Understanding the urgency of the situation, I wanted to find out right away if more could be done to help Erin save her baby and also protect Erin's own health. But whom could I call so late at night?

We had long been personal friends with pro-life attorney Colette Wilson and her husband, Tim. Colette had helped with the adoptions of babies saved from abortion through LifeSavers Ministries and other organizations, and the Wilsons themselves adopted babies who were saved from abortion. I decided to call the Wilsons to see if they had any ideas on what could be done. Tim suggested calling Dr. George Delgado, whom the Wilsons knew personally. Considering I was calling so late at night, I was relieved when Dr. Delgado answered the phone.

Dr. Delgado's medical clinic was called Culture of Life Family Services, and he often cared for women who had previously miscarried their babies and wanted to prevent future miscarriages. Dr. Delgado had found that progesterone was effective in preventing threatened miscarriages, so he hypothesized that it could be possible to use the same procedure to save a baby from the abortion pill.

However, he needed to find a doctor in Texas to treat Erin. Initially, the closest doctor he found was in Phoenix, many hours away from Erin. Fortunately, Dr. Delgado soon located Dr. Jonnalyn Belocura in Texas. Dr. Belocura had a supply of progesterone and was willing to see and treat Erin, using the dosage suggested by Dr. Delgado. All this was done at no cost to Erin, through the assistance of Dr. Delgado, Dr. Belocura, and LifeSavers Ministries.

Several weeks of progesterone shots presented no difficulty for Erin, and everything about the rest of her pregnancy was normal and healthy. Nevertheless, she continued to worry about whether the abortion pill had caused unseen harm to her baby. Part of Planned Parenthood's scare tactics had included an unfounded warning that her baby could have birth defects because of the abortion pill.

When her daughter, Kayley, was finally born, Erin was thrilled to see that she was perfectly healthy! Erin's mother, who continued to allow Erin and her daughter to live in her home, cherished her granddaughter from the moment she first saw her, even though she had advised Erin to abort her.

Erin continued to be apprehensive about raising a girl, because she feared that the negative cycle she had experienced with her own mother would repeat, causing future scars in Kayley's heart, but Erin's fears were never realized. Kayley has always been close to Erin, even when Erin confessed to Kayley that she was saved from abortion.

"I think that is beautiful because I have nothing to hide from her. God has broken that cycle in my life", Erin proclaimed. "Being transparent helps break those generational things that happen to us. She's the love of my life!"

I had lost touch with Erin during her pregnancy, but after Kayley was born, Erin called to share the good news and to thank us. I was overjoyed—not just about Kayley's life and health but also because Erin's pregnancy had been healthy and normal.

By the time Kayley was a toddler, Erin had found a good job. Eventually, she was able to afford her own house. "God is faithful, and God will provide", Erin says. "I'm able to have a better life, not living in regret, not living in darkness, but living in light and in the fullness that God has for me and my daughter." Erin also became a local ministry leader for an international Christian ministry, and she has served as a worship and prayer leader in her local church.

In the years that followed, I received calls from others who wanted to save their babies from the abortion pill, and several times I was able to connect these women with Erin so that they could hear firsthand about how their babies could be saved.

One of those women, who lives in New Jersey, had taken the abortion pill because she felt overwhelmed, being the mother of seven boys. But an internet search led her to me, the mother of eight boys, and seeing a photo of me with my eleven children, the woman decided to save her youngest, who turned out to be her only daughter. She continues to cherish her daughter, who is about two years younger than Kayley.

Erin and I are still close friends to this day, and we have visited each other many times over the years. "What can we do in the future to save more babies?" Erin asks. "I hope we can provide more help to women who have no support person, who feel like they are being forced into aborting their babies. I hope my testimony will give other women the courage to stand for what they know is right in their time of crisis. Abortion is a lie from hell that the enemy brings against women", Erin says today. "God knows what we need, even before we ask. He knows the plans He has for us even before we are born. He knows what we are called to do. But the enemy comes to steal, kill, and destroy. Life is a gift from Jesus, and only He can take it away."

23

The First Doctor to Be Banned from Saving Lives

By Dr. Dermot Kearney

On a Tuesday evening in late March 2021, I received a WhatsApp message from a nurse in the United States representing the Abortion Pill Rescue Network (APRN) hotline. She had received a call for help from a young mother in the United Kingdom who had taken the first abortion pill, mifepristone, earlier that afternoon and regretted doing so. She now wanted to try to save her baby. The nurse asked me whether I could help. She provided the contact details for the young lady, and within five minutes I was speaking with her on the phone. She was nineteen years old and was living in the English midlands.

Victoria (not her real name) was seven weeks and three days pregnant, which had been confirmed by ultrasound three days earlier. She was a university student, and her boyfriend had abandoned her because she was pregnant. Victoria had taken mifepristone four and a half hours earlier that day but regretted doing so immediately afterward. Fortunately, she had good support from her mother and brother, who helped her find the APRN website and hotline.

Victoria had been pressured by her family doctor and later by a psychiatrist who tried to convince her that she was not ready to be a mother and that having a baby at her age would destroy her life. They tried to convince her that her baby was merely tissue and that abortion was her best option.

Following our detailed conversation about APR treatment using progesterone, Victoria was determined to proceed with the rescue treatment to try to save her baby. The problem was that it was already 9:30 P.M. when the initial call for help had been received, and there was difficulty finding a local, late-night pharmacy open in her region that might also stock progesterone medication. Fortunately, we managed to find a pharmacy that was open until midnight, located forty-eight kilometers (thirty miles) away, and had micronized progesterone capsules in stock. The pharmacist was happy to accept an initial email prescription with the promise that the original signed prescription copy would be posted to him on the following day.

A prescription for micronized progesterone—Utrogestan 100 mg capsules—was transmitted with the standard dose regimen of 400 mg twice daily for three days to be followed by 400 mg once daily for a further fourteen days, if all was going well. The aim was to continue this treatment up to thirteen weeks' gestation if Victoria remained well and her baby remained alive. Victoria's mother drove her to the pharmacy, and she was able to commence the progesterone rescue treatment that night, approximately seven hours after she had taken the mifepristone tablet.

Victoria had some difficult moments with some light bleeding and mild cramps over the next five days, but these worrying symptoms resolved with continuing progesterone therapy. Her repeat ultrasound scan, performed nine days after commencing progesterone, revealed the wonderful news that her baby was alive and well with a strong heartbeat. She subsequently gave birth to a beautiful baby boy in early November 2021. With very good family support and the help of APR, a happy outcome was achieved in this case.

This case is just one of more than seventy that illustrate how APR operates in the United Kingdom. While coercion is not a prominent feature in all such chemical abortion cases, it unfortunately happens very often and is a major reason why some mothers opt to abort their children.

The number of abortions carried out in the United Kingdom has risen steadily in recent years, especially since 2016. This is largely due to the increasing availability of the abortion-inducing drugs mifepristone and misoprostol. In 2022, there were more than 250,000 abortions carried out in England and Wales alone.[1] In 2024, there were 18,710 in Scotland, which has more current statistics.[2] The abortion-inducing pills have been available in the United Kingdom since 1990. Until 2014, the majority of abortions were still surgical, whether by suction aspiration, dismemberment, or feticide and delivery. Since 2014, the numbers of drug-induced abortions have exceeded the numbers of surgical abortion procedures. About 86 percent of abortions in the United Kingdom in 2022 were carried out by drugs rather than by surgical procedures.[3]

While all abortions are gravely unjust, the one positive aspect of drug-induced abortion is that there is a window

---

[1] "Abortion Statistics, England and Wales: 2022", Office for Health Improvement and Disparities, updated April 9, 2025, https://www.gov.uk/government/statistics/abortion-statistics-for-england-and-wales-2022/abortion-statistics-england-and-wales-2022.

[2] "Termination of Pregnancy Statistics: Year Ending December 2024", Public Health Scotland, May 27, 2025, https://www.publichealthscotland.scot/publications/termination-of-pregnancy-statistics/termination-of-pregnancy-statistics-year-ending-december-2024.

[3] "Abortion Statistics, England and Wales: 2022".

of opportunity to save a baby if a mother changes her mind about proceeding with the abortion, even after she has taken the first abortion pill, mifepristone. This is the basis for the APR service. In surgical abortion, once the deadly instrument is introduced, there is no going back, but with chemical abortions, many babies can be saved with prompt and effective APR rescue treatment.

The story of the APR services in the United Kingdom began in 2014. Jack Scarisbrick, the cofounder of Life, a prominent British pro-life organization, which was formed after the passing of the Abortion Act in 1967, attended a council meeting of the Catholic Medical Association (CMA) UK in November 2014 with a request and a challenge.

Young mothers were approaching his organization, seeking help after taking the first abortion pill, mifepristone, and now wanting desperately to save their babies. He had heard reports from the United States that some babies had been saved by the prompt administration of progesterone therapy as long as the second abortion pill, misoprostol, had not been ingested.

The CMA council members were not aware of the possibility of APR using progesterone at that time. Many questions were raised relating to the number of mothers seeking this service, the possible efficacy of the APR treatment, and, particularly, the safety aspects of the progesterone protocol. Could babies really survive with the help of this treatment, and if they survived, was there a likelihood of significant congenital problems following exposure to mifepristone in early pregnancy? We agreed that we would investigate further, although there were not much data concerning APR at that time.

A major step forward occurred in May 2016 when another prominent pro-life leader, Clare McCullough, attended the CMA Annual Conference. She was founder of the pro-life Good Counsel Network based in London. She informed the CMA that more and more young mothers were coming to her organization seeking help to save their babies after regretting they had taken mifepristone. She pleaded with the CMA to join her in helping these young mothers. By that time, more information about APR, particularly in relation to efficacy and safety, had become available. As the newly elected president of the CMA, I promised Clare that the CMA would try to establish an APR program in the United Kingdom.

In September 2018, I attended the US CMA Annual Education Conference in Texas and met with Dr. George Delgado and other pioneers of APR in the United States. Dr. Delgado had recently published a landmark paper in a peer-reviewed medical journal on the success and safety of progesterone for APR following mifepristone.[4] I read this paper and other accounts of the APR experience in the United States. By that point, it was becoming very clear that APR using progesterone was very effective and very safe. I had noticed that opposition to the practice of APR was growing among the more extreme abortion advocates, particularly among those who had a vested interest in promoting chemical abortion.

A very important and influential article by Ruth Graham, entitled "A New Front in the War over Reproductive Rights: Abortion-Pill Reversal", was published in the *New York Times Magazine* in July 2017. It was a well balanced article with views expressed by both advocates and opponents of APR. I was particularly impressed by a statement attributed to Dr. Harvey Kliman, director of the

---

[4] George Delgado, Steven J. Condly, Mary Davenport, Thidarat Tinnakornsrisuphap, Jonathan Mack, Veronica Khauv et al., "A Case Series Detailing the Successful Reversal of the Effects of Mifepristone Using Progesterone", *Issues in Law & Medicine* 33, no. 1 (2018): 3–14.

Reproductive and Placental Research Unit at the Yale School of Medicine. He was quoted as saying, "I think this [APR using progesterone following mifepristone] is actually totally feasible." Kliman has published research on progesterone and miscarriage and is pro-choice on the issue of abortion. The article went on to say that "if one of his daughters ... had somehow accidentally taken mifepristone during pregnancy,... he would tell her to take 200 milligrams of progesterone three times a day for several days, just long enough for the mifepristone to leave her system." He concluded, "I bet you it would work."[5]

Following the second appeal for help by Clare McCullough and with the wealth of new and reassuring information, the CMA, at the council meeting in November 2018, decided it was time to establish an APR service in the United Kingdom. We wrote to National Health Service (NHS) England, the Royal College of Obstetricians & Gynaecologists (RCOG), and the Royal College of General Practitioners (RCGP) explaining the rationale and evidence for APR. We hoped that these bodies would be encouraged to introduce APR as part of mainstream medical practice in the United Kingdom.

The responses, however, were very negative and disappointing. The reply from the RCOG was the most disappointing and hypocritical. They stated that they did not support the use of "off-licence" (off-label) medications, acknowledging that progesterone is a licensed medical product but is not specifically licensed for abortion pill reversal. We replied by reminding them that misoprostol, the second drug used to induce abortion, is not licensed for that

[5] Ruth Graham, "A New Front in the War over Reproductive Rights: 'Abortion-Pill Reversal'", *New York Times Magazine*, July 18, 2017, https://www.nytimes.com/2017/07/18/magazine/a-new-front-in-the-war-over-reproductive-rights-abortion-pill-reversal.html.

use, although the RCOG had recommended it for that purpose. In addition, they encouraged the use of methotrexate in the medical management of ectopic pregnancy although it is not licensed for that indication.

Having received no replies to our second letters sent to each of the above-mentioned organizations, we then wrote to the General Medical Council (GMC), the main medical practitioner regulatory authority in the United Kingdom. We asked the GMC a specific question: "How should a doctor react if a pregnant woman has taken the first abortion pill, mifepristone, but then changes her mind before abortion has occurred and asks a doctor to help her save her baby?"

The GMC responded by stating that they do not provide any clinical advice, as it is not within their remit to do so. They referenced their guidance on Good Medical Practice and advised that all patients are entitled to be informed of all reasonable management options that are available to address their health-care needs. In addition, all patients are entitled to withdraw consent and to change their minds about continuing treatment or continuing interventions at any stage during any course of medical management. This advice was reasonable and encouraged us in the CMA to proceed with establishing an APR service within the United Kingdom, as we were satisfied that the evidence supporting APR, in terms of safety and efficacy, was very convincing. The APR service in the United Kingdom, with two doctors initially providing the service, began with the first cases in May and June 2020. In the first ten months, thirty-two babies' lives were saved as a result of their mothers seeking and accessing APR—until the APR service was temporarily disrupted in late April 2021.

On April 28, 2021, the two doctors providing the APR service, Dr. Eileen Reilly and I, received emails from the

GMC, informing us that complaints about our APR service had been forwarded to the GMC from a leading abortion provider, Marie Stopes International (also known as MSI Reproductive Choices) and from the RCOG. Allegations of potential professional misconduct had been received and were considered serious enough to warrant investigation. We were both ordered to attend a formal hearing under the auspices of the Medical Practitioners Tribunal Service (MPTS) on May 12, 2021.

Of note, I had already presented a report at a formal GMC Equality, Diversity, and Inclusion Strategy Forum meeting in early April 2021 on the CMA's involvement in providing an APR service to women within the United Kingdom. As the representative of the CMA on that forum, I delivered a report on various CMA activities over the previous months, and it included a summary of our APR activities. The report included the number of mothers requesting treatment and the number of babies already saved. The GMC chairperson at that meeting thanked me for the report. There was no mention of any complaints made to the GMC about CMA members providing an APR service, and there was no suggestion that the actions of doctors involved were already under investigation or that an investigation into possible professional misconduct might be necessary.

I had also delivered a presentation on the APR service to an all-party UK Parliamentary Committee meeting in early March 2021. That meeting was attended by several members of Parliament and several peers from the House of Lords. The report was enthusiastically received by all the attendees.

Unknown to me and Dr. Reilly, an orchestrated complaint and investigation into our APR service had already been initiated in January 2021. At that time, complaints were submitted to the GMC by MSI International and by the RCOG, in addition to a complaint led by a pro-abortion activist organization, ironically known as openDemocracy.

Ten specific complaints were made against me, and these were fully endorsed by the GMC. In brief, these allegations were made against me:

1. I remotely prescribed an unlicensed medication without evidence-base.
2. I did not liaise with abortion providers as the primary caregiver.
3. I denied patients opportunity to seek independent counseling.
4. I enforced personal beliefs on vulnerable patients.
5. I arranged ultrasound scans privately to conceal possibility of fetal abnormalities.
6. I gave money for medications and scans and arranged childcare.
7. I caused distress and delay in patients obtaining abortion care.
8. I acted outside my area of competence.
9. I did not follow NICE guidelines on abortion provision.
10. I failed to suitably consent patients and to maintain suitable medical records.

Needless to say, there was no evidence to support any of the allegations, with the exception of the ninth. It was true that I "did not follow NICE guidelines on abortion provision". I was not attempting to provide abortion. I, like Dr. Reilly, was responding to mothers who wanted to avoid having an abortion after they had taken the first abortion-inducing pill. It was very disappointing that the GMC was prepared to endorse all these false allegations without making any effort to determine whether there might be any evidence to support them. Both Dr. Reilly and I were summoned to attend an MPTS hearing on May 12, 2021. At that time, we had to inform the APR Network and all UK-based pro-life organizations what had happened and that we would not be able to continue the UK APR service.

Within two days, I received support from Christian Concern and their legal team, Christian Legal Centre, who offered free legal support. Through their wonderful chief executive officer and founder, Andrea Williams, they were determined to fight for justice. Within three days, an expert witness had been found who was prepared to consider the facts of the case.

We attended the MPTS hearing on May 12, 2021. Despite the lack of any evidence to support the allegations that had been made, the tribunal found that the allegations were serious enough to warrant a full investigation, and conditions were imposed upon my medical practice and that of Dr. O'Reilly. The main condition imposed upon me was that I "must not prescribe, administer, or recommend progesterone for abortion pill reversal treatment". In addition, I was not allowed to do any voluntary or private medical work without written permission from the GMC. The overall effect was that I would not be allowed to provide the APR service to any mother who wanted to save her baby after she had taken mifepristone and regretted doing so. I thereby became the first doctor in history to be actively banned from saving lives. Dr. O'Reilly became the second doctor to be banned from saving lives when similar conditions were imposed upon her later that same day.

These conditions were initially imposed for a period of eighteen months (the maximum time allowed for such a sentence) and would be reviewed at that stage and at six-month periods thereafter if considered necessary. Of note, the GMC actually demanded that we should both be suspended entirely from practicing medicine for a period of eighteen months, the maximum penalty that could have been imposed at that stage. The tribunal felt that such a penalty would be disproportionate, as neither of us had any record of previous concerning behavior and there had been no previous complaints made against us. Nevertheless, the conditions imposed, preventing us from offering help to mothers in desperate need, were very disappointing and frustrating.

We knew that witness statements from the mothers who had requested APR would be a key factor in determining the outcome of the case. In addition to a supportive expert witness statement, we quickly obtained ten witness statements from some of the mothers who had approached me seeking help with APR. Some were from mothers who had already given birth to their babies; some were from mothers who had a successful response and were due to have their babies in the near future. Some statements came from mothers who had commenced APR but unfortunately suffered miscarriage when the APR treatment was unsuccessful. We even obtained statements from two mothers who had decided not to proceed with APR and went ahead with the induced abortion but who now regretted doing so. We could have obtained many more such supportive witness statements, but my legal team decided that ten would be sufficient. We submitted these statements as evidence to the GMC.

We were subsequently very pleased to be told that a new hearing would take place on August 3, 2021, because new evidence had come to light. This hearing was convened three months earlier than had been planned as a result of the new evidence obtained on our side. Those who had brought a case against us had not yet produced any evidence to support the allegations they had made, nor would they. This hearing had been requested by our side. We therefore presumed that a favorable outcome was very likely. We were dismayed at the outset of the hearing, however, when the chairperson announced that no evidence would be examined, as the role of this "interim order tribunal" was not to verify the facts but merely to consider the seriousness of the allegations. This essentially rendered the August hearing a waste of time, as the conditions imposed in May were upheld. At that stage, my legal team made the decision to apply to the High Court on the basis that the penalties imposed upon me were unfounded and unjust.

After applying to the High Court in late September 2021, we were granted a hearing that would take place on February 24, 2022. In the meantime, we were informed by the GMC that they were still having difficulties trying to find an expert witness to support the cases against Dr. O'Reilly and me. Eventually they managed to find an expert witness in December 2021. When their expert witness reports were released in January 2022, they were favorable toward the APR service that we had been offering. The only concern expressed related to financial assistance that I had provided to some of the mothers seeking APR, to help them pay for their progesterone therapy when necessary and to help with payment for private ultrasound scans if there were difficulties obtaining early scans through the normal NHS channels. Once we were able to demonstrate that I was not actually paying the mothers or attempting to bribe them but that the payments were to the pharmacies and to the ultrasound service providers respectively, the concerns raised were effectively addressed.

We were preparing our case to proceed with the planned High Court appearance on February 24, when I received a telephone call from my legal representative on February

18 to inform me that the charges against me had been dismissed by the GMC. Some minutes later, I received an email from the GMC formally confirming this good news.

When the official Case Investigator's report was released, it concluded that there was no prospect of finding any evidence to support the allegations of professional misconduct that had been made against me. Consequently, the GMC made a recommendation to the MPTS that the case should be dismissed and that the conditions (sanctions) previously applied in May 2021 should be revoked. The conditions were formally revoked some days later. Interestingly, the conditions imposed upon Dr. Reilly were not revoked until two months later. Presumably, the GMC had no reason to rush a revocation recommendation in her case, as there was no High Court threat proceeding from her legal representatives. She had been represented by a secular medical defense organization and not by the Christian Legal Centre, by her own choice.

Since March 2022, APR service for mothers and their children in the United Kingdom has resumed. A valuable lesson learned from this entire experience is that the abortion industry relies upon the pro-life movement to be fearful and silent. The abortion industry is built upon lies and fear. These, however, are very unstable and shaky foundations. When challenged with the expression of truth and with courage, the abortion industry has no rational answer. Above all, they fear the courage of pro-life advocates. They are fearful that the general public will be made aware of the truth about abortion.

As of early 2025, we know of at least seventy babies who have been saved in the United Kingdom as a result of their mothers reaching out and seeking APR support, after regretting taking the first abortion-inducing pill, mifepristone. We know that many others would have been saved if it had not been for the unjust campaign initiated by the abortion industry and endorsed by the GMC that prevented us from offering the APR service to women in the United Kingdom for a period of almost twelve months.

We hope and pray that many more lives will be saved with this continuing service. There is an urgent need to create greater awareness that APR is available and that it is safe and effective in saving lives. We need more doctors, nurses, and pharmacists to be aware of the service and to have the willingness and courage to provide the service to mothers who desperately seek our help.

In my own personal experience in providing APR, I have so far received a total of 148 requests for the treatment (as of March 2025) from mothers who regretted that they had taken mifepristone and now wanted to try to save their babies. From this cohort of 148 requests, 94 mothers (64 percent) decided to proceed with the rescue treatment. The other 54 (36 percent), for various reasons, decided not to commence treatment, or it was too late to do so. Some may have represented fake calls from journalists or pro-abortion supporters seeking information about the APR service, although many were genuine calls from mothers in distress who wanted to save their babies but were under pressure from others to proceed with abortion. Many of these mothers who decided not to commence APR contacted me later, after they had undergone abortion, to express their gratitude for the offer of help and for the explanation of APR. Many expressed regret that they did not proceed with progesterone rescue therapy.

Of the 94 who commenced treatment, at least 7 stopped treatment and subsequently proceeded to abortion. In each case, their decision to abort was made under coercion from others, usually boyfriends or husbands. Of the remaining 87 mothers who started and seemed to continue with the APR treatment, 13 subsequently stopped responding to messages of support. The outcomes for these mothers and their babies are unknown. They may have decided to proceed with abortion or may have suffered later miscarriage. They may have given birth to healthy children and simply didn't want to be reminded of the terrible choice they had originally made by taking mifepristone before seeking APR.

Of the initial 148 mothers who contacted me about receiving APR, 74 who commenced and continued rescue treatment have a known outcome. To date, 33 babies have been born to mothers who contacted me for APR help. There have been 25 confirmed failures, where miscarriage occurred within fifteen days of commencing and continuing APR treatment. Some later miscarriages occurred, well past fifteen days after APR had commenced. It is not known if these were natural miscarriages or if they resulted from mifepristone and may therefore represent APR failure. There were at least 7 cases of initial success with APR and continuing pregnancy well after the fifteen-day period after commencing APR, but they were subsequently lost to follow-up. It is possible that these may represent additional successful responses to APR. In one case, the pregnancy was ectopic, which was discovered through the ultrasound scan arranged after the mother had commenced APR. The progesterone was not continued, and the mother received successful conservative management.

The overall success rate for APR in the United Kingdom in terms of live births and likely successful outcomes is 50–55 percent. If the later miscarriages are considered to be successful, the APR success rate may be even higher. The success rate could be as high as 63 percent if the unknown outcomes that had progressed past fifteen days of APR treatment are considered to have been successful. The failure rates could be as low as 40 percent if the unknown cases that had progressed past fifteen days of treatment are considered successful but could be as high as 50 percent if strictly measuring confirmed failures versus live births and likely live births to come.

When discussing APR using progesterone, I always emphasize that if a mother takes both abortion pills, mifepristone and misoprostol, in early pregnancy, there is a 98–99 percent certainty that her baby will die. If she takes the first abortion pill, mifepristone, but doesn't take the second abortion pill, misoprostol, and doesn't receive rescue treatment with progesterone, there is an 80 percent chance that her child will die. There is therefore a 20 percent chance her child may survive, even without APR treatment, as long as she doesn't take misoprostol. If she takes the first abortion drug, mifepristone, but does not take misoprostol and receives high-dose progesterone rescue treatment promptly and continues the treatment for at least two weeks, there is a 50–55 percent chance that her baby will survive to birth. This is an astonishing success rate. There are very few interventions in medicine whereby a certain mortality rate of 80 percent can be consistently reduced to a less than 50 percent mortality rate by the application or administration of a simple, inexpensive medical treatment. Abortion pill reversal with progesterone is truly one of the great advances in medicine over the last fifty years.

Regardless of how many babies' lives are saved and how many mothers are helped, the APR service is worthwhile. Sometimes there is a temptation to become despondent when the APR treatment is unsuccessful and miscarriage occurs. Such news can be heartbreaking. I have discussed this with my colleague, Dr. Eileen Reilly, many times. She reminds me that providing the service is worthwhile even if only one life is saved. We both agree that in our many years working as medical professionals, the APR service is the most rewarding work we have ever done.

Part 3

24

Common Themes

I have had many conversations with abortion pill reversal colleagues about common threads we see running through the many APR cases in which we have had the privilege to assist. While no cases are exactly alike, certain themes do seem to recur. When I was reviewing the testimonials for part 2 of this book, this idea was definitely reinforced.

The first theme is that those who eventually choose APR often have misgivings or at least ambivalence about choosing chemical abortion. In their stories, you can sense the inner struggle and turmoil. It often is not perceived as picking between two options; rather, abortion is felt to be the only solution—albeit a bad one—to a huge predicament.

Many are crying when they take the abortion pill. In Cynthia's account, she related that she ran out of the abortion center before returning and taking the pill. Another woman shared that she was clutching the mifepristone pill in her hand, crying and trying to decide what to do, when the doctor sternly told her to take it because it would otherwise melt in her clenched hand.

In a way, the woman in a crisis pregnancy sees herself as boxed in a corner, with abortion the only way out. I have often felt that it is quite analogous to suicide. Few, if any, people choose suicide as a positive action. No, they are desperately suffering and feel the only way to ease the psychological pain is to end their lives. Some people who have survived suicide attempts have shared that they felt immediate regret after attempting to take their lives. The difference with abortion, of course, is that instead of taking her own life, the mother takes that of her preborn baby.

In Sarah's testimonial, she shared the heart-wrenching letter she wrote to her preborn baby. In it, she expressed her love and apologized for what she was doing. She asked for God's forgiveness. It sounds very much like a suicide letter. However, this "suicide" would be reversed.

The second common thread is related to the first: immediate or nearly immediate regret. Often, women start to search on the internet about reversing the abortion soon after taking the mifepristone, sometimes in the abortion center parking lot. The regret is often accompanied by a moment of clarity for these women. Some instantly realize they have done something wrong, something violating their core principles, something that needs to be stopped and reversed.

Less often but still commonly, women waver after seeking information on reversal. The people and factors that influenced them to choose abortion do not magically vanish. The pressures to abort are still felt, sometimes even after starting the APR therapy. APR doctors, nurses, and counselors always offer support, insight, and solutions. However, they only propose, never impose, always respecting the autonomy of the women, even when they choose to continue with the abortion.

Third, many of the women we have helped had unstable support systems at the onset. In a recent study of 880 women who chose APR, only 14 percent were married.[1] Many were having sex in uncommitted relationships, even casually.

---

[1] George Delgado et al., manuscript in peer review.

On the other hand, we have seen that those who chose APR eventually had at least one strong support person. Most had several people cheering for them. My late mother-in-law used to wisely say, "You only need one friend in life." Having that one person who believes in you and will be an anchor makes all the difference in the world.

Fourth, as can be seen in the testimonials, most of those who chose APR had some religious foundation or background. When the going got very tough, they knew they could lean on God. Their faith often saved them and their babies.

Fifth, when many women first crystallized their regret, they called the center where they received their mifepristone because they did not know where else to turn for help. We have heard some consistently similar anecdotes from women about what they were told when they first called their abortion centers asking whether they could stop their chemical abortions.

Many were told these things, quite erroneously:

- "You have to finish what you have started."
- "Your baby is sure to have birth defects."
- "Reversal does not work."
- "You signed a paper saying you would take the second drug [misoprostol]."

Employees at these abortion centers are either lying or have not kept up with the medical literature. In fact, there is strong and increasing medical evidence that APR is safe, both for the mom and baby (no increased risk of birth defects), and effective.

The last common theme is gratitude. I have not heard of a single mom who has regretted reversing her chemical abortion with progesterone. In fact, the nearly unanimous response is one of pure joy and appreciation. In all my years of practicing medicine, including delivering babies and caring for the dying, the greatest gratitude that has been expressed to me has come from the mothers, fathers, and family members of APR babies. There is no regret with APR, only faith, hope, and love.

25

What's in a Name?

Names can be more than simple words we use to refer to people. Oftentimes, parents put a great deal of thought into a baby name, hoping that the name might provide context, a hint of mission, and a structure for the child. Sometimes, children are named after parents, family members, ancestors, famous personages, or virtuous people.

In ancient times, names had even more importance. Names clearly suggested or determined the roles people would fill in God's plan, family destinies, and the lives of others. The circumstances of people's lives and births often helped determine their names. The names were an expression of appreciation for what God had done for them or the good fortune that had befallen them.

For example, Moses means "drawn out of the water"; he was pulled from the Nile River by Pharaoh's daughter.[1] Judah means "praise".[2] The book of Numbers tells us that when the Israelites were in the desert for forty years and would break camp, Judah would go first.[3]

Sometimes, God would change people's names when there was a shift or elevation of mission. Abram became

---

[1] Ex 2:10.
[2] Gen 29:35.
[3] Num 2:9.

Abraham,[4] and Sarai became Sarah.[5] In the New Testament, Jesus gave the apostle Simon a new name, Cephas[6] (rock), which comes to us in English as Peter, when He declared He would build His Church with him as the foundation.

In the Christian era, it has been common to name babies after great saints. The idea was that the child might emulate the virtues of the saint and that the particular saint might become a patron, someone who would constantly intercede before God for the person.

Many of us who are involved with abortion pill reversal have been impressed by the names that some parents of APR babies have chosen. Many are rich in meaning and extremely thoughtful. The names are often biblical in origin. Many have direct allusions to God and His love for us.

Of course, I am unaware of the names of the vast majority of the thousands of babies saved by APR. However, I would like to share some of the names of which I am aware and that seem to have special meaning. Some of the special meanings may not be what the parents intended. However, in some ways, that is what makes names so rich—they may have unforeseen interpretations apart from what the parents imagined.

Names of APR Babies

Mariam is the Aramaic and Arab form of Mary (Miriam in Hebrew), the name of the mother of Jesus. Miriam was also the name of the sister of Moses. The different forms of the name are very popular across all three monotheistic religions, Christianity, Judaism, and Islam. Mary was a

[4] Gen 17:5.
[5] Gen 17:15.
[6] Mt 16:18.

great example to us when she gave her fiat, her statement of acceptance of God's plan for her, even though she did not understand the plan. Many APR mothers and fathers have chosen life, even when they did not understand the whys and the hows of what would come.

Ezekiel means "God strengthens".[7] Ezekiel was one of the major prophets of the Old Testament. The book of Ezekiel was written at the time of the Babylonian exile to chastise and encourage the people of God. One mom specifically chose this name because she felt God gave her the strength and courage to choose to save her baby's life.

The name Christian speaks for itself; it means "follower of Christ". One dad chose that name for his son to declare unequivocally his mission. Another baby was likewise named as a follower of Christ; her name is Chrystyanna.

Zechariah means "God remembers".[8] In naming her baby Zechariah, the mom wanted to acknowledge that God never forgot her, even when she strayed from His path.

In the Gospel of Luke, we learn that Zechariah was the father of John the Baptist. Like APR parents, Zechariah was given a second chance. When he doubted the angel Gabriel, who declared to him that his elderly wife, Elizabeth, would bear a son, he was struck mute.[9] Later, going against the expectation of naming his firstborn son after himself, he followed God's plan and named him John (Jonah). Once he had obeyed, his tongue was loosed, and he began to speak.[10]

Zechariah was also the name of a minor prophet in the Old Testament. His prophesies in the postexile Holy

---

[7] "Ezekiel Meaning", Abarim Publications, accessed March 29, 2025, https://www.abarim-publications.com/Meaning/Ezekiel.html.

[8] "Zechariah Meaning", Abarim Publications, accessed March 29, 2025, https://www.abarim-publications.com/Meaning/Zechariah.html.

[9] Lk 1:8–20.

[10] Lk 1:63–64.

Land encouraged the Jews to rebuild the temple that had been destroyed by Nebuchadnezzar, the king of the Chaldeans.[11] Rebuilding the destroyed temple is somewhat analogous to the rebuilding, or reversal, that takes place with APR. Both Zechariahs were priests in the line of Aaron and thus had special roles in worship and in atoning for the sins of God's people.

Elizabeth was the mother of John the Baptist, a cousin of Mary, and the wife of Zechariah. Her name means "God is an oath."[12] Against all odds, Elizabeth conceived in her old age. Against all odds, mothers exercise their second chance at choice and attempt to save their babies with APR treatments.

Isaiah means "God is salvation."[13] It has similar etymological roots to the name Yeshua. Isaiah was a major Old Testament prophet whose message was one of conversion. Many of his passages prefigure or announce the coming of Emmanuel, God among us. APR is a process of conversion and certainly one of salvation.

Jesus was chosen as the name for at least one APR baby. Although the name is not commonly used in non-Spanish-speaking countries, in Spain and Latin America it has long been popular. The Hebrew version of Jesus is Yeshua, which means "God saves." Thus, the name given to Jesus as prescribed by the angel Gabriel fit Him to a tee. APR saved the modern-day child named Jesus and thousands of babies from abortion.

Eden is the name of the garden God created for Adam and Eve where, until the Fall, they lived in perfect harmony with Him and each other. Perhaps the APR baby

---

[11] Zech 6:9–15.

[12] "Elizabeth", Behind the Name, accessed March 29, 2025, https://www.behindthename.com/name/elizabeth.

[13] "Isaiah", The Bump," accessed March 29, 2025, https://www.thebump.com/b/isaiah-baby-name.

Eden was so named as a reminder that God can restore all things, even when we make terrible decisions.

Eliana means "my God has answered."[14] The APR mom may have been expressing her gratitude for the second chance at choice.

Hannah was mother of the prophet Samuel, the last judge of Israel and the one who anointed both King Saul and King David. Hannah suffered from infertility and over many years repeatedly asked God to give her a son. After she conceived and bore Samuel, she presented him for God's service, and the first book of Samuel records her beautiful canticle, where she rejoices for what God has done for her.[15] The Magnificat of Mary in Luke's Gospel is structured in a similar fashion to the Canticle of Hannah.[16] The name Hannah means "favor" or "grace".[17] It is clear that graces flow through APR and through the baby named Hannah.

Elijah (English) and Elias (Spanish) mean "the Lord is God."[18] Elijah was one of the greatest prophets in the Old Testament; in fact, he appeared with Moses at the Transfiguration, representing all the prophets. The mere reality of babies born because of APR is a prophetic message.

Jordan means to "flow down" or "descend".[19] The Jordan River is arguably the most famous river in the world. In both ancient and modern times, it holds high religious, geographical, economic, and agricultural significance.

---

[14] Rebekah Wahlberg, "Eliana", BabyCenter, accessed March 29, 2025, https://www.babycenter.com/baby-names/details/eliana-6205.

[15] 1 Sam 2:1–10.

[16] Lk 1:46–55.

[17] "Hannah", SheKnows, accessed March 29, 2025, https://www.sheknows.com/baby-names/name/hannah/.

[18] Keshia Roelofs, "Elijah", The Bump, accessed March 29, 2025, https://www.thebump.com/b/elijah-baby-name.

[19] Emily McNamara, "Jordan", The Bump, accessed March 29, 2025, https://www.thebump.com/b/jordan-baby-name.

Opposite Jericho, Joshua led the Israelites across the Jordan into the Promised Land. Christians see this crossing as a prefigurement of baptism, when Christians cross into a new promised land. It was in the Jordan River that John baptized Jesus. The APR baby Jordan crossed into a new promised land when her life was snatched from the jaws of death.

Zlatan is a Slavic name that means "gold".[20] Gold is a symbol of wealth and royalty. Edward is another name related to wealth, meaning a "wealthy guardian".[21] Both Zlatan and Edward were given the riches of life when they were saved from abortion by APR.

In the Old Testament, Noah built the ark to save a remnant of mankind from the chastisement of the Flood. The name means "rest" or "peace".[22] Imagine that, peace among death, similar to APR.

Ember's mom said that she picked the name because God did not allow her to be burned out. The fire now burns brightly.

Santiago is a Spanish name that is translated to Saint James in English. It is a composite name: *Sant* means "saint" or "holy", while *Iago* is a derivation of Jacob (in Latin, *Iacobus*). Two apostles were named Jacob, likely a common Hebrew name in those times. The name Jacob means "supplanter".[23] Baby Santiago was given the opportunity to supplant death. At least one APR baby is named Diego, which was derived from the name Santiago. Diego

---

[20] "Zlatan", Ancestry, accessed March 29, 2025, https://www.ancestry.com/first-name-meaning/zlatan.

[21] "Edward", Ancestry, accessed March 29, 2025, https://www.ancestry.com/first-name-meaning/edward.

[22] Avril Whelehan, "Noah", The Bump, accessed March 29, 2025, https://www.thebump.com/b/noah-baby-name.

[23] "Jacob", Ancestry, accessed March 31, 2025, https://www.ancestry.com/first-name-meaning/jacob.

of Alcala became a saint in his own right; the city of San Diego is named after him.

Evelyn is an interesting name with different meanings and interpretations. It likely was derived from the Norman French name Aveline, and as you might expect, it has been linked to the name Eve, our first mother in Genesis. A common meaning is "desired".[24] This APR baby will always know she was loved and desired, for her mother courageously changed course to save her life.

Leo in Latin means "lion".[25] A lion's heart has long been a symbol of courage, of fighting with great fortitude. In the book of Revelation, Jesus is called the Lion of Judah. In the fifth century, Saint Leo the Great was pope and courageously maintained Christian unity and orthodoxy. Perhaps he is most famous for meeting Attila the Hun as he prepared to conquer Rome. Against all odds and with great courage, Leo convinced him to leave.[26] The APR movement is filled with great examples of lionhearted heroes.

Maverick is a great name for an APR baby because many mothers have been mavericks, standing tall in spite of the pressure to continue their abortions from family, friends, and abortion center workers. The name means "nonconformist". It originated when people named their children after a Texas rancher, surnamed Maverick, who refused to brand his cattle the way all the other ranchers did.[27]

In Israel, a mother named her APR daughter Hallel, which means "praise" in Hebrew. She picked the name

---

[24] Wendy Wisner, "Evelyn Name Meaning", December 17, 2024, Parents, https://www.parents.com/evelyn-name-meaning-origin-popularity-8627694.

[25] "Leo", Behind the Name, accessed June 13, 2025, https://www.behindthename.com/name/leo.

[26] Jared Zimmerer, "Attila the Hun, Leo the Great, and the Battle of Wills", Word on Fire, November 10, 2017, https://www.wordonfire.org/articles/fellows/attila-the-hun-leo-the-great-and-the-battle-of-wills/.

[27] Grace Royal, "Maverick", Nameberry, May 8, 2025, https://nameberry.com/b/boy-baby-name-maverick.

because she feels it was a miracle her baby was saved from abortion.[28] The name expresses her gratitude by praising God.

Ella is a name with many possible origins and manifold meanings. Sources I checked indicated it can mean "other", "goddess", "pistachio tree", "bright one", and "light". It may have independently been derived from Ancient Hebrew, Modern Hebrew, Greek, Spanish, English, and German.[29] Ella has great depth of meaning, just as APR has depth of meaning. Each APR baby is a bright one who bears the light of the intrinsic value of each and every human person. While no APR baby is a goddess, each and every one is made in the image of God. Pistachios are mentioned in the Bible when Israel instructs his son to take them as a gift to the Egyptian ruler, whom they did not yet know was Joseph.[30] Pistachios were highly valued in the ancient Middle East. Legend has it that King Nebuchadnezzar included pistachio trees in the Hanging Gardens of Babylon. Also, it is reported that Queen Sheba delighted in pistachios.[31]

Sawyer is an English name that derives from the word "saw" and means someone who works with wood.[32] The

---

[28] Brooke Myrick, "Abortion Pill Reversal Turns the World Upside Down", *Pregnancy Help News*, April 3, 2025, https://pregnancyhelpnews.com/abortion-pill-reversal-turns-the-world-upside-down.

[29] "Ella", Baby Names, Mama Natural, accessed April 16, 2025, https://www.mamanatural.com/baby-names/girls/ella/; "Ella", Bounty, accessed April 5, 2025, https://www.bounty.com/pregnancy-and-birth/baby-names/baby-name-search/e/ella; Ruchelle Fernandes, "Ella Meaning and Origin", First Cry Parenting, January 16, 2023, https://parenting.firstcry.com/articles/ella-name-meaning-and-origin/.

[30] Gen 43:11.

[31] "Pistachios Are Mentioned in the Old Testament in Genesis 43:11", *South Florida Reporter*, February 25, 2020, https://southfloridareporter.com/pistachios-are-mentioned-in-the-old-testament-in-genesis-4311/.

[32] "Meaning of the First Name Sawyer", Ancestry, accessed April 6, 2025, https://www.ancestry.com/first-name-meaning/sawyer.

connection that came to my mind is to history's most famous carpenter, Joseph, the foster father of Jesus.

Names are more than mere identifiers. Some of the names chosen by APR mothers and fathers for their babies have great depths of meaning. They have given us a glimpse into the struggles, triumphs, fears, and trust that are interwoven in these powerful stories.

26

David Versus Goliath: Why Big Abortion Doesn't Want You to Know About APR

As I discussed in chapter 5, abortion is a big business, to the tune of hundreds of millions of dollars in the United States. Not only that, but it is a linchpin in the liberal agenda and ideology. Therefore, it should not be a surprise that a large web of interconnected organizations and powerful individuals protects Big Abortion. I call it the Medical-Abortion Complex. This complex has at its foundation Planned Parenthood, the National Abortion Rights Action League (NARAL), and other abortion activist groups. It includes mainstream medical organizations like the American College of Obstetricians and Gynecologists (ACOG), the American Medical Association, and the American Academy of Family Physicians. They are bolstered and defended by the American Civil Liberties Union (ACLU) and deep-pocketed liberal organizations and individuals. Open Society Foundations, the group funded by George Soros, is in the mix. Many feel that US government agencies such as the Food and Drug Administration (FDA), National Institutes of Health (NIH), and United States Agency for International Development (USAID) are biased in favor of and protect abortion. The FDA regulates drugs, while the NIH funds research.

Abortion supporters have been critical of abortion pill reversal since the early days. Before long, a massive echo chamber of repeated, irrational criticism was created. The articles in mostly progressive publications repeat the same misinterpretations, distortions, and lies about APR. The mainstream media have been part of the echo chamber too.

I was initially surprised that so many leaders of the Medical-Abortion Complex were vehemently opposed to APR. They called themselves "pro-choice". Why did they oppose a second chance at choice? Why did they not want women who changed their minds to have access to and information about APR? Were they really pro-choice or simply pro-abortion?

Dr. Donna Harrison, a well-respected pro-life obstetrician-gynecologist, researcher, and expert on mifepristone told me one day, "You poked the bear." She was right: APR was perceived as a serious ideological threat by the Medical-Abortion Complex. The bear was annoyed and ferociously fought us.

A few abortion researchers have been especially critical of APR. Daniel Grossman, MD, is a clinician and researcher at University of California, San Francisco (UCSF) and the associated Bixby Center. He also has been a leader at Ibis Reproductive Health. Both Bixby and Ibis are known as abortion and contraceptive colonists. They seek to transplant Western-style liberal views and programs of contraception and abortion to developing countries.

Fortunately, many traditional, family-friendly countries, nearly all of them developing countries, have been fighting the imposition of a pro-abortion agenda. The battle of ideologies was manifest at a November 2024 meeting at the United Nations marking the thirtieth anniversary of the International Year of the Family, according to an article by Stefano Gennarini. The brave poorer countries were able to have the wording "reproductive health", which is code for abortion services, removed from the final resolution. "While traditional countries were elated by the outcome, Western countries were bitterly disappointed that the resolution did not include abortion language or recognition of homosexual couples as families", according to the article.[1]

Lest you think the aggressive United Nations support of abortion is not pervasive, see another article by Gennarini from 2025. In it, he writes, "The UN working group on discrimination against women and girls claims that governments have an international obligation to force all hospitals to provide abortions, including religious hospitals. The report goes as far as describing institutional conscientious objection as 'impermissible' and a 'human rights violation' ".[2] What some might think unimaginable is occurring: A UN group is advocating that pro-life doctors and hospitals, even those based on religion, be compelled to offer abortions.

Dr. Grossman was an author of an article in the journal *Contraception* that sought to support the false narrative that if a woman takes mifepristone and then changes her mind, she should just wait and see and not take progesterone to reverse the chemical abortion.[3] The errors in

---

[1] Stefano Gennarini, "Brave African Delegates Fight Abortion in Landmark UN Family Resolution", C-Fam, November 21, 2024, https://c-fam.org/friday_fax/brave-african-delegates-fight-abortion-in-landmark-un-family-resolution/.

[2] Stefano Gennarini, "UN Group Says Government Must Force Medical Personnel to Provide Abortions", C-Fam, January 16, 2025, https://c-fam.org/friday_fax/un-group-says-government-must-force-medical-personnel-to-provide-abortions/.

[3] Daniel Grossman, Kari White, Lisa Harris, Matthew Reeves, Paul D. Blumenthal, Beverly Winikoff et al., "Continuing Pregnancy After Mifepristone and 'Reversal' of First-Trimester Medical Abortion: A Systematic Review", *Contraception* 92, no. 3 (2015), https://doi.org/10.1016/j.contraception.2015.06.001.

that article were thoroughly exposed by my colleague Dr. Mary Davenport in her landmark article in 2017.[4]

Amanda Marcotte, in an article on the *Slate* website, stated, "Grossman says that the progesterone probably won't hurt a woman if she's under medical supervision, but he's concerned that the advertising of this procedure could mislead the public about the prevalence of abortion regret."[5] That answered the question for me that I had asked since APR was first criticized so vehemently. The reason Big Abortion attacks APR so aggressively is because they know if the public sees that women regret starting their chemical abortions and seek to reverse them, that calls into question the pro-choice narrative that abortion is a great good for all women. If it were such a great good, why would some regret it?

Speaking of abortion regret, the Medical-Abortion Complex has long insisted that women rarely regret their abortions. They also say that women rarely change their minds after taking mifepristone. To support those assertions, they rely on biased and poorly designed studies that utilized the Turnaway cohort data. The Turnaway data were gathered and analyzed by a group called Advancing New Standards in Reproductive Health (ANSIRH), a UCSF group directed by Dr. Grossman. Multiple studies have used the same flawed Turnaway data to conclude that women do not regret their abortions. David Reardon published an article in a peer-reviewed journal showing

---

[4] Mary Davenport, George Delgado, Matthew P. Harrison, and Veronica Khauv, "Embryo Survival After Mifepristone: Review of the Literature", *Issues in Law & Medicine* 32, no. 1 (2017): 3–18.

[5] Amanda Marcotte, "The Newest Crisis Pregnancy Center Offer: 'Abortion Reversals'", *Slate*, December 8, 2014, https://slate.com/human-interest/2014/12/abortion-reversals-the-latest-anti-abortion-offer-from-crisis-pregnancy-centers.html.

that only 31 percent of the women invited to be in the Turnaway study agreed to join and half of the 31 percent dropped out before completing the study. Additionally, the question about regret required a simple yes or no answer; no shades of gray were allowed.[6]

On the other hand, the research by Reardon had a high participation rate and used 11 visual analog scales in order to capture nuanced responses. In the study, "33% described their abortions as Wanted, 43% as Inconsistent, 14% as Unwanted and 10% as Coerced. In addition, 54% answered mostly affirmative ($\geq$50) to the statement that they would have continued their pregnancy if they had more financial security, 42% would have given birth if they had more support from others, and 60% reported they would have preferred to give birth if they had received either more emotional support or had more financial security."[7] As you can see, only a third of those surveyed really wanted their abortions, and more than 60 percent would have continued their pregnancies if they had more support from others. This study totally shatters the false narrative that women rarely regret their abortions.

The Creinin Study

Dr. Mitchell Creinin is a professor at UC Davis and the director of the Complex Family Planning Fellowship. Complex Family Planning is a newer subspecialty in obstetrics and gynecology that was started at least in part to

---

[6] David C. Reardon, Katherine A. Rafferty, and Tessa Longbons, "The Effects of Abortion Decision Rightness and Decision Type on Women's Satisfaction and Mental Health", *Cureus*, May 11, 2023, https://doi.org/10.7759/cureus.38882.

[7] Ibid.

teach doctors how to perform third-trimester abortions. Dr. Creinin has had a consultative relationship with Danco Laboratories, the first US company to market mifepristone.

Dr. Creinin designed a study that he hoped would discredit APR. Speaking about his proposed study in a National Public Radio online interview, he said, "I want to own that", referring to his quest to disprove APR.[8]

He conducted a double-blind, placebo-controlled, randomized trial comparing our high-dose oral progesterone protocol to placebo.[9] What exactly does that mean? *Placebo-controlled* means that there is a group in the study whose participants receive a pill or substance that visually resembles the active treatment medication but has no active ingredient. *Randomized* means that participants are randomly assigned to either the active treatment or placebo group; they do not have a choice. In general, when there is a placebo group, the participants are "blinded", which means they do not know whether they are receiving active treatment or placebo.

From a purely scientific standpoint, the study design checked all the boxes; it met the gold standard. Although it was stopped early, the study was published in the prestigious journal *Obstetrics and Gynecology*, first online in December 2019.

Unfortunately, from a life perspective it was unethical. All the preborn babies would be killed: Those in the placebo group would be killed by the abortion pill, and those whose

---

[8] Mara Gordon, "Controversial 'Abortion Reversal' Regimen Is Put to the Test", NPR, March 22, 2019, https://www.npr.org/sections/health-shots/2019/03/22/688783130/controversial-abortion-reversal-regimen-is-put-to-the-test.

[9] Mitchell D. Creinin, Melody Y. Hou, Laura Dalton, Rachel Steward, and Melissa J. Chen, "Mifepristone Antagonization with Progesterone to Prevent Medical Abortion: A Randomized Controlled Trial", *Obstetrics & Gynecology* 135, no. 1 (2020): 158–65, https://doi.org/10.1097/AOG.0000000000003620.

mothers received progesterone would eventually be terminated by surgical abortion—a double-jeopardy situation.

Pregnant women seeking abortion who presented to an abortion center in Sacramento, California, were asked to join the study. Those who agreed were randomized by a computer to one of two groups, the progesterone group (our APR protocol) or the placebo group (no treatment to reverse the abortion). All of them received mifepristone first.

In the article, Dr. Creinin gave credence to our research by citing and utilizing our statistics. He used the high-dose oral progesterone protocol from our 2018 study.[10] In order to calculate how many patients he would need in the two arms of the study, he borrowed Dr. Mary Davenport's figure of 25 percent survival of preborn babies exposed to mifepristone if no APR treatment is offered.[11]

His pretrial statistical calculations indicated he would need forty total patients in order to generate what is called "statistically significant data". What does that mean? Imagine you wanted to prove your hypothesis that when a coin is flipped, 50 percent of the time it lands heads and 50 percent of the time tails. Would you do four flips to prove your point? Probably not—you might by chance get three of one and one of the other. Would you do a million flips? That would likely be excessive. A pretrial statistical analysis would allow you to predict how many coin flips you would need to generate numbers you could trust.

Dr. Creinin stopped his study after twelve patients were enrolled because of "safety concerns". Three women called

---

[10] George Delgado, Steven J. Condly, Mary Davenport, Thidarat Tinnakornsrisuphap, Jonathan Mack, Veronica Khauv et al., "A Case Series Detailing the Successful Reversal of the Effects of Mifepristone Using Progesterone", *Issues in Law & Medicine* 33, no. 1 (2018): 3–14.

[11] Davenport et al., "Embryo Survival After Mifepristone," 3–18.

911 and were transported to emergency departments. The after-study spin was that APR is unsafe and should not be recommended.

However, looking at Dr. Creinin's own words in the article leads us to a much different conclusion. He wrote, "First, patients who receive high-dose oral progesterone treatment do not experience side effects that are noticeably different than placebo." Remember, placebo is an inactive pill, no drug.

Of the three women who went to the emergency room, one had been given progesterone; she was in the group that received abortion pill reversal treatment. She panicked because of the bleeding that followed her chemical abortion and unsuccessful reversal. In the emergency department, "no intervention was needed", according to Dr. Creinin. In other words, she did not need to be there. That patient outcome was no reason to stop his study.

The other two women were both in the placebo group; they had received mifepristone but not progesterone. Both required emergency surgical suction abortions in the emergency department to control bleeding. One of them also required a blood transfusion. In the abstract of the article, Dr. Creinin stated, "Patients in early pregnancy who use only mifepristone may be at high risk of significant hemorrhage."

Dr. Creinin's study supported the safety and effectiveness of using progesterone to reverse mifepristone abortions. Because he enrolled only twelve patients instead of the planned forty, the data did not reach statistical significance. However, the numbers are telling, nonetheless.

Per the article, "Overall, four of six patients in the progesterone group and two of six patients in the placebo group had continuing pregnancies at 2 weeks. Excluding the two patients who did not finish treatment, these rates are four of five and two of five, respectively." In other words, looking at all twelve patients, the abortion reversal rate using progesterone was 67 percent (4 out of 6) and the reversal failure rate was 33 percent (2 out of 6). If the two that voluntarily left the study are excluded, the reversal rate was 80 percent (4 out of 5) and the failure rate was 40 percent (2 out of 5). These numbers are in the same ballpark as our published data.[12]

I have been perplexed by the number of patients Dr. Creinin intended to enroll in the study. His pretrial analysis predicted he would need forty patients, twenty in each group. It is very common for studies such as this to enroll more patients than the predicted number in case the pretrial calculations underestimated the needed sample size or patients exit the study early due to side effects, relocation, death unrelated to the study (such as in a motor vehicle accident), and other reasons. However, in the abstract, he wrote, "We planned to enroll 40 patients ..." Was not enrolling excess patients a way to guarantee that statistical significance would not be achieved?

The true conclusions from the Creinin study support the effectiveness of using progesterone to reverse mifepristone abortions and show that using progesterone was not associated with risks. Even an attempt to disprove APR added to the evidence for it.

An FDA Chokehold

After the publication of our first two APR studies, my intention was to conduct a randomized controlled trial. The first two studies were retrospective reviews—good

---

[12] Creinin et al., "Mifepristone Antagonization with Progesterone", 158–65; Delgado et al., "A Case Series," 3–14.

science but not the highest level of scientific inquiry. The gold standard is considered a randomized placebo-controlled study.

Early on, we realized that as ethical researchers, we could not have a placebo group in our randomized controlled trials. The preborn baby of a mother receiving placebo would be doomed to death. No mother desperately wanting reversal would accept the possibility of placebo (see chapter 27 for the CPR analogy).

Although we could not and would not conduct placebo-controlled APR studies, we felt we could design trials that were controlled and randomized. Instead of comparing active treatment with placebo, we would compare different types of active treatment to each other.

With that in mind, I reached out to a respected researcher at a major medical school in the United States. He was very interested and thought that a randomized controlled trial would be important. Additionally, he shared my opinion that a placebo group would be unethical.

In September 2020, we submitted the proposed study protocol to the university's institutional review board (IRB). The IRB, sometimes called an ethics panel, is an important part of research on human subjects. Its main purpose is to ensure the safe and ethical treatment of study subjects. We were expecting that there would be some back-and-forth communication and negotiation with the IRB—that's part of the process of approval. What we did not expect was the IRB compelling us to submit an investigational new drug (IND) application with the FDA.

Our active treatment study drug, progesterone, is in no way a new drug. In fact, it has been safely used in pregnancy for over fifty years. Unfortunately, the IRB staff wanted us to request a new official indication for progesterone in its use for APR.

An official indication would be useful in that the package insert that comes with the progesterone would include information on using progesterone for APR and the statement of approval by the FDA. However, the IND application to the FDA would be an extra bureaucratic layer and would slow the study. In fact, not only did it slow the study, but it froze it for years.

We were perplexed and concerned regarding the university's insistence on the FDA application. Were there people at the university, within or outside the IRB, who were trying to sabotage the study? On the other hand, were the IRB members simply being extremely cautious because of the now radioactive nature of APR research? Was it simply poor judgment on the part of the IRB? Could it be a combination of these reasons? Perhaps we will never know.

The result was that the FDA now had full control of the destiny of the study protocol we submitted. In October 2020, we requested that the FDA provide us with a waiver of the IND application process. About ten days later, they responded with a clear no. The FDA was requiring a full application.

It was not until February 2021 that the university filed the study application on our behalf with the FDA. About a month later, the FDA responded by telephone that the study had been put on a full clinical hold. That meant we could not launch the study until the FDA gave us the green light. We were in their clutches.

In late April 2021, the FDA sent a detailed letter. There were twelve major "hold" points—issues that had to be resolved for the study to move forward. After extensive discussions with members of our team, the university, and outside consultants, we completed a revised protocol and compiled responses to the FDA objections. All this information was sent to the FDA in August 2021.

In September 2021, representatives of the university had a telephone conversation with the FDA. The FDA representative stated that there were still unresolved issues. A letter was promised by October 8. On October 7, the university received an email stating that there would be a short delay in the FDA's response.

By December 2021, we still had not received the promised reply from the FDA. We were now over a year into the project, and the study was nowhere near starting. Finally, in mid-January 2022, the FDA responded again by email to tell us that many people needed to give input. My suspicion was that we were getting extra scrutiny at the FDA, perhaps by people who were philosophically opposed to APR. That January communication included a reminder that we could not legally launch the current study protocol. The official letter responding to our modifications was still pending.

On April 5, 2022, the FDA issued a Continue Clinical Hold letter. On July 15, 2022, our team responded to the letter, offering possible solutions and modifications so that we could start the study. The FDA essentially ignored us after that letter, which was sent about a year and a half after our initial application. For two and a half years, this US government agency, which is funded by our tax dollars and is supposed to be impartial and fair, ignored an extremely important and timely study proposal. There was radio silence until we requested a Type A meeting with them in October 2024. At that point, it had been over four years since we had submitted the protocol to the university IRB and three and a half years after our FDA application was submitted.

In early December 2024, we had our Type A meeting with representatives of the FDA. I was surprised and interested to hear that the head of the division who was handling our application would be part of the teleconference. The meeting did not resolve the issues causing the delay to our study, but it went somewhat better than expected. Although the FDA representatives did not apologize for the lengthy silence, they did acknowledge it and took responsibility for it.

Earlier in our back-and-forth with the FDA, they insisted that we have a comparator group called an "expectant management" group—a group of women who took mifepristone but not misoprostol and did not take progesterone reversal treatment. We had stated that we felt that not offering APR treatment to some of the study subjects (that is, doing nothing) would be unethical. Also, from a practical standpoint, how would we convince women who had called the APR hotline, seeking APR, to join a study where they might not receive treatment to save their preborn babies?

Furthermore, in an early letter to the FDA, we had questioned why they were requiring us to have a control group when they had approved mifepristone itself for chemical abortion without a randomized study and without a control group (see chapter 4). The FDA did not address the inconsistency and continued to insist that testing of the unique life-saving treatment would require a control group. That is, preborn babies would have to die.

One of the FDA doctors in the meeting said we simply had to tell the subjects that APR is unproven, that there is no evidence supporting its effectiveness. That doctor felt that if we simply told them, they would believe us. Essentially, she was directing us to deceive the subjects, since we do have evidence that APR is effective.

As a compromise, we had offered to track patients who went to abortion centers seeking mifepristone chemical abortions but for whatever reason never took the second drug and never sought APR—that is, women who still wanted abortions but never took the second drug. In the meeting, the FDA refused that option.

During the meeting, it was clear to me and others that the FDA doctors and staff did not believe that APR is effective. They totally discounted the five studies in the medical literature that all support the effectiveness and safety of APR. They even said that we could not compare different progesterone treatment protocols until we first compared progesterone treatment with expectant management. It felt as if they were baking in conditions that would either make the study impossible or doom it to failure.

Big Tech: Big Block

Mark Zuckerberg, Facebook founder, CEO of Meta, and self-styled architect of the metaverse, admitted that Facebook had censored information that contradicted the orthodoxy as defined by the US government, the CDC, and the World Health Organization in regard to COVID-19. Big Tech willingly or under pressure from the US government went along with filtering the narrative, trying to manipulate the information that the general public was allowed to hear.

This same censorship by Big Tech, the gatekeeper of social media, has also occurred with APR. In 2021, Live Action was running very successful Google ads informing women about the possibility of APR. An abortion-rights activist group called Center for Countering Digital Hate issued a "report" that was later promulgated by *The Daily Beast* and other platforms alleging that APR is unsafe.[13] On what did they base that? Their misinformation was based on the dishonest spin and the misinterpretation of data from the Creinin study.

---

[13] Leah Savas, "Censoring Pro-Life Choice: Big Tech Companies Ban Live Action's Abortion Pill Reversal Ads", World, September 21, 2021, https://wng.org/roundups/censoring-pro-life-choice-1632236192.

In a press release, Lila Rose, the president of Live Action, stated, "In a dramatic and unprecedented move, Google has sided squarely with extremist pro-abortion political ideology, banning the pro-life counterpoint and life-saving information from being promoted on their platform. They aren't hiding their bias anymore: Google's censorship baldly reveals that the corporation is in the pocket of the abortion industry."[14]

According to Prolife Across America, "Facebook and Microsoft Ads have declined many of our online ads, and Google will intentionally bury us in search engine results." Furthermore, the group asserts, "We were effectively canceled by a major outdoor advertising company that has a monopoly on [b]illboards in many cities. After being an established client for many years, new management suddenly categorized us as an 'advocacy group' and mandated a rate of 2–3 times *more* than our non-profit rate."[15]

Senator Josh Hawley wrote to Google CEO Sundar Pichai in 2022, "I am concerned that, in the name of providing 'clarity' in search results, your company is deliberately limiting pregnancy resource centers' outreach efforts. By doing so, Google has joined the far left's campaign to punish pregnancy resource centers, following the Supreme Court's ruling in *Dobbs v. Jackson Women's Health Organization* earlier this year."[16]

---

[14] Noah Brandt, "Google Censors and Suppresses Life-Affirming Messages", Press Release, Live Action, September 14, 2021, https://www.liveaction.org/bigtechcensors/.

[15] "Our Ads Under Attack; We Need Your Help!" Prolife Across America, accessed April 7, 2025, https://prolifeacrossamerica.org/our-ads-under-attack-we-need-your-help/.

[16] "Hawley Demands Answers from Google on Apparent Efforts to Punish Pregnancy Resource Centers," Senator Josh Hawley, September 23, 2022, https://www.hawley.senate.gov/hawley-demands-answers-google-apparent-efforts-punish-pregnancy-resource-centers/.

In 2021, eleven other US senators wrote to Google expressing their concern about Google's censorship of Live Action's ads promoting the Abortion Pill Reversal hotline. "While banning pro-life APR ads, Google continues to allow ads for purveyors of the deadly abortion pill *mifepristone* by mail, despite the fact this drug has resulted in at least 24 mothers' tragic deaths and at least 1,042 mothers being sent to the hospital. Google's double standard on abortion is disingenuous and an egregious abuse of its enormous market power to protect the billion-dollar abortion industry."[17]

An in-depth probe by Carole Novielli connects the dots, and with the Medical-Abortion Complex, there are always plenty of dots, many with familiar names. The basis for Google's censorship was a report by the Center for Countering Digital Hate. The report cited a group called openDemocracy as a source for its claims about APR. That group is funded by "the David and Lucile Packard Foundation, which invested $14.2 million into Danco's startup in 1996 and is now also investing millions into GenBioPro, Inc., an FDA-approved company which began manufacturing a generic version of the abortion pill in 2019".[18] Danco was formed as a single-drug pharmaceutical company to sell mifepristone in the United States (see chapter 2).

The George Soros groups, Open Society Foundations, and the Rockefeller Foundation, all linked to promoting abortion in the past, have been funders of openDemocracy,

---

[17] Steve Daines to Sundar Pichai, September 16, 2021, https://www.daines.senate.gov/wp-content/uploads/imo/media/doc/9.16.2021%20Google%20Abortion%20Pill%20Reversal%20Ad%20Letter.pdf.

[18] Carole Novielli, "Group That Asked Big Tech to Ban Abortion Pill Reversal Ads Took All Its Claims from Pro-Abortion Sources", Live Action, September 19, 2021, https://www.liveaction.org/news/ban-abortion-pill-reversal-ads-sources/.

according to Novielli. The ACOG is also listed as a source of information for the report attacking APR. The ACOG has received funds from abortion supporter Ibis Reproductive Health, which in turn is funded by Danco. The David and Lucile Packard Foundation has also directly given money to Ibis.[19]

The ACOG received $1.4 million from the Buffet Foundation—hundreds of thousands per year for several years, according to the Live Action report. Not surprisingly, Buffet was one of the first Danco investors.[20]

In 2023, US Representative Jerry Carl called out Google Maps in an op-ed. Without notification, Google removed Capitol Hill Pregnancy Center, a pro-life pregnancy help center, from its search service. Carl declared, "Woke corporations have been getting away with silencing conservative voices and values for a long time, and I have had enough."[21] Google later reinstated the listing and claimed that it was "incorrectly removed", according to a Live Action article by Gabriela Pariseau on December 20, 2023.[22]

Many years ago, the playing field was made less level when the Associated Press, which publishes its manual of guidelines called *The Associated Press Stylebook*, directed journalists not to use the terms *pro-life* or *pro-lifers*. On the other hand, they allowed the self-chosen term *pro-choice* for those who support abortion. The term *pro-life* had been in

---

[19] Ibid.

[20] Ibid.

[21] US Rep. Jerry Carl, "Rep. Carl: Demanding Accountability for Big Tech Censorship of the Pro-Life Movement", Yellow Hammer, December 5, 2023, https://yellowhammernews.com/rep-carl-demanding-accountability-for-big-tech-censorship-of-the-pro-life-movement/.

[22] Gabriela Pariseau, "Lawmaker Pens Letter to Google CEO over Pro-Life Censorship", Live Action, December 20, 2023, https://www.liveaction.org/news/lawmaker-letter-google-pro-life-censorship/.

use since the early 1970s and has long been accepted in the pro-life community.²³

In 2013, Planned Parenthood began a retreat from one of its favorite terms, *pro-choice*. The retreat was probably because the euphemism lost its luster as many mentally made the automatic association between pro-choice and pro-abortion.²⁴ *The Associated Press Stylebook* later went along with Planned Parenthood's wishes and stopped suggesting the term *pro-choice*.²⁵

The Associated Press Stylebook has a powerful effect on journalists. In the last year, I asked a reporter to identify me as pro-life. She replied that her editors would not allow that because it would violate the stylebook's directives.

In a *Daily Signal* article by Virginia Allen and Mary Margaret Olohan, new guidelines by the stylebook were discussed. It says to "use the modifiers anti-abortion or abortion-rights; don't use pro-life, pro-choice or pro-abortion unless they are in quotes or proper names. Avoid abortionist, which connotes a person who performs clandestine abortions".²⁶ The mainstream media are in lockstep with the demands and desires of Big Abortion.

---

²³ Micaiah Bilger, "AP Tells Reporters to Never Use the Term 'Pro-Life'", LifeNews.com, July 12, 2017, https://www.lifenews.com/2017/07/12/ap-tells-reporters-to-never-use-the-term-pro-life/.

²⁴ Anna North, "Planned Parenthood Moving Away from 'Choice'", BuzzFeed, January 9, 2013, https://www.buzzfeed.com/annanorth/planned-parenthood-moving-away-from-choice.

²⁵ Kelly McBride, "How Abortion Language Evolves", NPR, April 4, 2024, https://www.npr.org/sections/publiceditor/2024/04/04/1242805450/how-abortion-language-evolves.

²⁶ Virginia Allen and Mary Margaret Olohan, "Major News Style Guide Tells Reporters 'Don't Use Pro-Life, Pro-Choice or Pro-Abortion,' Instead Say 'Anti-Abortion or Abortion-Rights'", *Daily Signal*, December 8, 2022, https://www.dailysignal.com/2022/12/08/major-news-style-guide-tells-reporters-dont-use-pro-life-pro-choice-or-pro-abortion-instead-say-anti-abortion-or-abortion-rights/.

As of 2024, about fifteen states had enacted laws requiring that information about the possibility of reversing mifepristone chemical abortions be given to women at abortion centers. Some of those laws are now inactive, mostly because the states no longer allow abortion. Other states attempted to pass similar laws. I testified before a Colorado state legislature committee and in a Tennessee lawsuit regarding an informed consent law.[27]

In almost all instances, these efforts simply to give women information on APR, not ban or restrict abortion, were met with aggressive legal action by groups such as the ACLU, Planned Parenthood, and mainstream medical organizations. Their actions support Dr. Grossman's opinion that allowing people to know that some women seek to reverse their chemical abortions "could mislead the public about the prevalence of abortion regret".[28] Of course, it is not misleading to acknowledge that women do, in fact, often regret their abortions. If they did not, then there would be no demand for APR. The facts speak for themselves. The bear has been poked and continues its vicious attack on APR.

---

[27] "State Laws and Policies: Medication Abortion", Guttmacher, April 23, 2025, https://www.guttmacher.org/state-policy/explore/medication-abortion.

[28] Marcotte, "The Newest Crisis Pregnancy Center Offer".

27

Answering Critics: Would You Ban CPR?

Abortion pill reversal (APR) is analogous to cardiopulmonary resuscitation (CPR). APR is a unique way to save the life of a preborn person, while CPR is a unique way to save the life of an already-born person. Both involve emergency, life-or-death scenarios. If no action is taken, death is very likely.

CPR was approved and gained wide acceptance without any randomized controlled scientific studies on humans. No one dared design a study comparing active CPR with sham treatment or expectant management—that is, doing nothing. Once we had good evidence that CPR was effective, conducting studies where some patients did not receive CPR would be unethical and would never be approved.

Imagine how utterly ludicrous it would be to conduct a study comparing CPR with no treatment. In such a situation, the code blue team in a hospital responding to a patient with cardiac arrest would first check a computer-generated list to see whether the patient should receive chest compressions and artificial ventilation. Likewise, paramedics in such a study would first check a computer to see whether the man who had gone down on the street was randomized to receive CPR or not.

External chest compressions were first tried in 1891 by a German surgeon, Dr. Friedrich Maass, in a successful attempt to save a child who had cardiac arrest related to anesthesia. Although his chest compressions were performed on the left side of the chest, not directly on the sternum, they were effective. He published his work in Germany and France. However, the breakthrough was forgotten and never gained traction.[1]

Modern CPR on humans was first described in a July 9, 1960, article by Dr. William Kouwenhoven and associates, of Johns Hopkins Hospital.[2] They used their knowledge of chest compressions gleaned from animal studies and from earlier versions of resuscitations in humans to develop modern chest compressions with and without mouth-to-mouth or mouth-to-nose ventilations. Besides describing some animal experiments, the rest of the landmark article was a series of case reports, similar to our first APR article in 2012.

Once the 1960 CPR article was published, word spread about the effectiveness of the procedure and more doctors tried it. By 1970, physician leaders in Seattle led by cardiologist Dr. Leonard Cobb of the University of Washington embarked on an ambitious program to educate tens of thousands of laypersons in the techniques of CPR. In the first two years, the widely successful program had trained one hundred thousand people.[3]

---

[1] Richard L. Taw Jr. "Dr. Friedrich Maass: 100th Anniversary of 'New' CPR", *Clinical Cardiology* 14, no. 12 (1991): 1000–1002, https://doi.org/10.1002/clc.4960141211.

[2] W. B. Kouwenhoven, James R. Jude, and G. Guy Knickerbocker, "Closed-Chest Cardiac Massage", *JAMA* 173, no. 10 (1960): 1064–67, https://jamanetwork.com/journals/jama/article-abstract/328956.

[3] "History of CPR", American Heart Association, accessed April 8, 2025, https://cpr.heart.org/en/resources/history-of-cpr.

None of the developments depended on randomized controlled trials in humans. Everyone knew, and knows today, that a study that did not offer treatment to all subjects would be unethical.

CPR is not the only example of an effective treatment being utilized even if it has not been scrutinized by gold standard studies. Exceptions are made when a treatment has no alternative, treats a serious or life-threatening condition, and is assumed to be safe.

Such conditions exist for APR. There is no alternative to progesterone therapy for the reversal of mifepristone abortions. An initiated chemical abortion is certainly a life-threatening situation for the preborn baby. Furthermore, the mother seeking reversal desperately wants to save her preborn baby. Progesterone has been used safely in pregnancy for over fifty years,[4] and the safety data of at least five published studies are very reassuring.[5] Nonetheless,

---

[4] G. Dante, V. Vaccaro, and F. Facchinetti, "Use of Progestogens in Early Pregnancy", Facts, Views and Vision, ObGyn 5, no. 1 (2013): 66–71.

[5] George Delgado and Mary Davenport, "Progesterone Use to Reverse the Effects of Mifepristone", Annals of Pharmacotherapy 46, no. 12 (2012), https://doi.org/10.1345/aph.1R252; George Delgado, Steven J. Condly, Mary Davenport, Thidarat Tinnakornsrisuphap, Jonathan Mack, Veronica Khauv et al., "A Case Series Detailing the Successful Reversal of the Effects of Mifepristone Using Progesterone", Issues in Law & Medicine 33, no. 1 (2018): 3–14; Deborah Garratt and Joseph V. Turner, "Progesterone for Preventing Pregnancy Termination After Initiation of Medical Abortion with Mifepristone", The European Journal of Contraception & Reproductive Health Care 22, no. 6 (2017): 472–75; Mitchell D. Creinin, Melody Y. Hou, Laura Dalton, Rachel Steward, and Melissa J. Chen, "Mifepristone Antagonization with Progesterone to Prevent Medical Abortion: A Randomized Controlled Trial", Obstetrics & Gynecology 135, no. 1 (2020): 158–65, https://doi.org/10.1097/AOG.0000000000003620; Joseph V. Turner, Deborah Garratt, Lucas A. McLindon, Anna Barwick, and M. Joy Spark, "Progesterone After Mifepristone: A Pilot Prospective Single Arm Clinical Trial for Women Who Have Changed Their Mind After Commencing Medical Abortion", The Journal of Obstetrics and Gynaecology Research 50, no. 2 (2024), https://doi.org/10.1111/jog.15826.

despite APR meeting the criteria I have outlined, naysayers continue to criticize our efforts and dismiss APR because of the lack of randomized controlled trials, except for the Creinin study (see chapter 26), which actually supports the safety and effectiveness of APR.

It should also be noted that mifepristone was approved in the United States without a randomized placebo-controlled trial (see chapter 4 for a detailed discussion).

Our critics also attack us for prescribing progesterone "off label". Off-label prescribing means using an FDA-approved medicine for a condition different from the one for which it was officially approved. Off-label prescribing is well accepted and commonly practiced; about 21–32 percent of all US prescriptions are off label.[6]

In obstetrics, three medications have been routinely used to treat preterm labor: magnesium sulfate, terbutaline, and nifedipine. None of the three has the FDA indication for stopping preterm labor. All are examples of the widespread off-label use of medications.

Additionally, it has been very common over the years for abortion pill prescribers to use mifepristone off label, especially by using it in pregnancies with gestational ages greater than the approved limits. They criticize us for what they have long done. The double standards abound.

---

[6] Gail A. Van Norman, "Off-Label Use vs Off-Label Marketing of Drugs", *JACC: Basic to Translational Science* 27, no. 8 (2023): 224–33, https://doi.org/10.1016/j.jacbts.2022.12.011.

28

Steno Institute

Just as I never thought I would be a pioneer in a revolutionary medical movement like abortion pill reversal nor a researcher publishing multiple scientific papers, I did not imagine that I would start a nonprofit institute. With APR and APR research, needs were present, and I was called to act, create, and generate.

When encouraging others, I often repeat the saying "God does extraordinary things with ordinary people." As time progressed, the adage became meaningful for me personally. God was working through me, an ordinary person, to accomplish some remarkable and beneficial things.

When Culture of Life Family Services (COLFS) transferred the APR Network to Heartbeat International in 2018, the COLFS board felt that aside from providing APR treatment to local patients, the organization should not have a primary role in the further evolution of APR. At the same time, Heartbeat did not want to be in the business of perfecting medical protocols. That left me with the assigned task of studying and perfecting APR. I knew that the science of APR was in its infancy and needed more research and development.

Knowing a thing or two about nonprofits due to my work at COLFS since 2005 and my association with a large nonprofit hospice, I felt confident in starting a new platform. At this time, the culture was becoming increasingly hostile to APR, and the field of play was not level. Funding for APR research would be difficult to find, some researchers might hesitate to study the controversial topic, and journals might balk at publishing papers on APR. A solid nonprofit that could promote, encourage, fund, and carry out APR research was badly needed. It would also have a role in the education of medical professionals and the general public. Increasing awareness and being a resource for policymakers and thought leaders would also be goals.

For the board of directors, I chose two extremely competent and ethical clinicians, Mary Davenport, MD, and Matthew Harrison, MD. Both had been involved with APR early in its development; in fact, Dr. Harrison had performed the very first reversal.

In choosing a name for the institute, I wanted a word or phrase that was easy to remember, intriguing, and meaningful. I had long been attracted to the concept of the complementary nature of faith and reason. Pope Saint John Paul II had written in *Fides et Ratio*, "Faith and reason are like two wings on which the human spirit rises to the contemplation of truth."[1] I believed that we needed strong science, rooted in reason, to develop APR. However, without faith, our ethical compass could run afoul. Science without ethics is like a river with no riverbanks, powerful but very dangerous. We must insist on strong ethical guardrails for all research and scientific advancement.

The elite club of contemporary science now unfortunately demands that its members check their faith at the door. Modern science, in many ways, has evolved into

---

[1] Pope John Paul II, *Fides et Ratio* (Pauline Books and Media, 1998), 7.

scientism. Scientism is the false belief that science and only science can answer all questions. The proposition of scientism is self-refuting.[2] That is because science makes assumptions of premises and order that it cannot prove. It relies on an internal order that can be explained only by the acknowledgement of a master designer.

Some have mused that, in discovery, science answers the what and the how, while religion answers the who and the why.[3]

I chose to name the nonprofit organization Steno Institute, after Blessed Nicolas Steno (Steensen in Danish, Stensen in English), a fine example of the blending of faith and reason to achieve excellence. He was highly distinguished as a humanitarian and a man of reason. The seventeenth-century Danish scientist, physician, and bishop was a truly gifted person who used his talents and abilities to further understanding in many areas of science as well as theology. Faith and reason were not at odds in his mind but were two halves of the same whole.

Blessed Nicolas is considered the father of modern geology and paleontology. He discovered laws and principles that explain why rock sedimentation occurs in layers (strata), and he has been called the Father of Stratigraphy. Blessed Nicolas first explained the concept of the formation of fossils. The idea came to him when he

---

[2] J.P. Moreland, "Why Strong Scientism Is Self-Refuting", J.P. Moreland, October 3, 2018, https://www.jpmoreland.com/2018/10/03/why-strong-scientism-is-self-refuting/.

[3] Yehuda Fogel, "Rabbi Jonathan Sacks at the Intersection of Science and Religion: A Tribute", 18Forty, November 19, 2020, https://18forty.org/articles/crossroads-of-science-religion-a-tribute-to-rabbi-jonathan-sacks/; Matt D'Antuono, "Science Answers What and How—Faith Answers Who and Why", *National Catholic Register*, August 22, 2019, https://www.ncregister.com/blog/science-answers-what-and-how-faith-answers-who-and-why.

was dissecting a shark's mouth and noticed how closely the teeth resembled "tongue stones", which were fossils of teeth.[4] In the last century, a mineral, Stenonite, was named after him.[5]

Additionally, he made groundbreaking discoveries in anatomy and medicine. He was the first to describe the heart as a muscle.[6] All of us carry his name since we each have two salivary gland ducts in our cheeks, which he first described and which are called ducts of Steno (or Stensen's ducts).

Blessed Nicolas underwent a religious transformation and conversion to Catholicism after observing a Eucharistic procession, while serving as a physician in Italy.[7] He ceased his medical and scientific pursuits and dedicated his life to theological study. Eventually he was made a bishop and was known for his piety. Blessed Nicolas kept an austere lifestyle as a bishop, including selling his bishop's ring to help the poor.[8] He set a superb example in his life by honoring the dignity of the least of our brothers and sisters. In his last discourse as a scientist, he said, "Beautiful is what we see. More beautiful is what we comprehend. Most beautiful is what we do not comprehend."[9]

---

[4] "Nicholas Steno", UC Berkeley, accessed April 10, 2025, https://ucmp.berkeley.edu/history/steno.html.

[5] Michon Scott, "Niels Stensen (Steno)", Strange Science, updated October 12, 2013, https://www.strangescience.net/stensen.htm.

[6] Alex Benjamin Shillito, "How the Heart Became Muscle: From René Descartes to Nicholas Steno", (PhD diss., University of South Florida, April 2019), https://digitalcommons.usf.edu/cgi/viewcontent.cgi?article=9136&context=etd.

[7] "The Scientist and Blessed Nicolas Steno", accessed April 10, 2025, https://judeatl.com/wp-content/uploads/2019/03/NicholasSteno_Flue_Lateau.pdf.

[8] "Bl. Nicolas Steno", Society of Catholic Saints, accessed April 10, 2025, https://catholicscientists.org/scientists-of-the-past/bl-nicolas-steno/.

[9] Ibid.

Blessed Nicolas refused to accept all scientific dogma at face value; instead, he chose to research matters himself.[10] This drive to seek truth and not to accept uncritically what the scientific community has proclaimed as orthodoxy inspires us to promote unbiased research supporting the dignity of human life. That is why Steno Institute exists.

In the short time of its existence, Steno Institute has promoted APR at various conferences and gatherings. It has helped fund the randomized controlled trial that, unfortunately, the FDA has stalled (see chapter 26). As of 2025, a large retrospective cohort study involving 880 patients is in peer review, and another study of patients being seen in a clinic in the Midwest is in the planning stages.

Additionally, Steno has helped fund the work of Stephen Sammut, PhD, who has developed a rat model of mifepristone abortion reversal (see chapter 3). Dr. Sammut has also collaborated on two Steno human studies, bringing his skills as a statistician.

The Steno motto is "life-affirming research". It leaves the horizon open to expanding into other areas of research in the pro-life arena. This is very important because of the huge bias that has been exposed in research around abortion, all part of the work of the Medical-Abortion Complex (see chapter 26).

One of our primary goals is to perfect APR protocols. We want treatments that are the safest and most effective. A secondary goal is to study the psychological factors involved when women choose to initiate chemical abortion and when they choose to reverse. Other areas of interest

---

[10] Chris Gaylord, "How Nicolas Steno Changed the Way We See the World, Literally", *Christian Science Monitor*, January 11, 2012, https://www.csmonitor.com/Technology/Horizons/2012/0111/How-Nicolas-Steno-changed-the-way-we-see-the-world-literally.

include the psychological effects that chemical abortion has on a woman. Few people give thought to how aborting a baby in one's own home might transform how that space is perceived in the future.

As the Steno mission has evolved, I appreciate even more the importance of increasing awareness about APR, which has been a multipronged and multilevel effort. First, we hope to inform women who might be in the situation of having taken mifepristone and wondering what they can do. If they feel regret, we don't want them to have to search long for help.

Second, we want to educate those who might be future friends, mentors, or acquaintances of women who might be seeking reversal. Well-informed people will give better counsel and be able to help women seeking reversal more quickly.

Third, we want to educate physicians and other medical practitioners about the safety and effectiveness of APR. We would like them to feel comfortable recommending APR and offering treatment if it is in their scope of practice.

Fourth, we want to inform influencers, those voices on social media who have such great sway with young adults. Many are not afraid to buck the mainstream message and will share stories and information about APR.

Fifth, we want to influence policymakers and government officials. Our people deserve fair laws, just regulations, and unbiased bureaucrats at the FDA, NIH, and health departments. They work for us; we deserve a fair shake.

29

The Future with APR as the Standard of Care

What will the future hold for abortion pill reversal? I am not naïve, and I realize that APR will always be controversial, just as offering pregnancy help services to women in crisis pregnancies is questioned by some. Offering assistance to others will often be criticized by those who feel that the help represents an ideological threat to strongly supported beliefs or practices. Such is the case with the Medical-Abortion Complex and abortion. For them, I suspect that no amount of evidence, no randomized controlled study, will ever be enough.

However, I am optimistic that those in the middle, those who are reasonable, those who are not heavily invested emotionally, academically, politically, or financially in abortion will come to accept the safety and effectiveness of APR. These are the physicians, other health-care practitioners, nurses, policymakers, and ordinary citizens who care about what is right and about the importance of giving women who want it a second chance at choice. These are the people who value life over ideology.

One of the reasonable people is Dr. Harvey Kliman, director of the Reproductive and Placental Research Unit at the Yale School of Medicine. "It makes biological sense", he told Ruth Graham in a *New York Times Magazine* article, when asked his opinion about APR. "I think this is actually totally feasible." According to Graham, Kliman "is in favor of abortion rights.... But if one of his daughters came to him and said she had somehow accidentally taken mifepristone during pregnancy,... he would tell her to take 200 milligrams of progesterone three times a day for several days, just long enough for the mifepristone to leave her system: 'I bet you it would work.'"[1]

Eventually, I think the bitter attacks against APR will soften as those who oppose it see that they are on the losing side of the argument, with more evidence accumulating to support the safety and effectiveness of APR. They will realize that most people will not buy into the rhetoric, hyperbole, and lies. The die-hard supporters of the Medical-Abortion Complex will likely still oppose APR, but I doubt they will devote as much energy to that opposition as they do now.

Currently other physicians and I are working on at least three different APR studies. More articles in the medical literature will solidify the evidence. With increased knowledge and understanding, our protocols will be even more effective.

The growth of social media and alternative news platforms will advance the acceptance of APR. More than ever before, people distrust the legacy media and look to alternative sources of information. More people are seeking to find information for themselves and coming to their own conclusions. The mainstream media and the Medical-Abortion Complex are no longer considered trustworthy. People now know better. Additionally, the

---

[1] Ruth Graham, "A New Front in the War over Reproductive Rights: 'Abortion-Pill Reversal'", *New York Times Magazine*, July 18, 2017, https://www.nytimes.com/2017/07/18/magazine/a-new-front-in-the-war-over-reproductive-rights-abortion-pill-reversal.html.

halo that Planned Parenthood once claimed has been removed as people discover the truth about this organization: that its profit is centered on abortion.

As public opinion emerges in favor of APR, I predict that emergency departments will become common sites of first contact. Ultrasound is readily available in emergency departments to confirm viability of the preborn exposed to mifepristone. The first dose of progesterone—oral, vaginal, or intramuscular—can be administered in the emergency department. Follow-up can be arranged with the patient's established primary care practitioner or her obstetrician, or she could be referred to another doctor for subsequent care.

I also foresee many women starting APR treatment with their own primary care practitioners or obstetricians. Any physician who treats women with threatened first trimester miscarriages is well equipped to offer APR. It is also a natural fit for family physicians, internists, pediatricians, and physicians who are available for patients' urgent and emergent medical needs. The many APR physicians whom I have had the privilege to meet universally say that helping women reverse their chemical abortions has been one of the most gratifying aspects of their careers.

30

Final Words

Abortion pill reversal has definitely been the climax and highlight of my medical career. Many doctors go into medicine for three reasons: to save lives, mitigate diseases, and alleviate suffering. Saving a life is by far the most gratifying and tangibly meaningful thing I can do as a physician. For family physicians and most doctors, concrete opportunities to save lives rarely present themselves. Usually, we are treating minor illnesses or struggling to manage chronic diseases like diabetes, obesity, or hypertension.

However, with abortion pill reversal, I have been able to save lives that would have otherwise been lost to abortion. I have seen and met children who are alive because of the assistance I gave to their mothers, who desperately sought a second chance at choice.

Not only has it been rewarding to save the preborn babies, but it has also been especially fruitful for me to work with brave mothers and fathers who not only sought to reverse their choices for abortion but also were striving to repair other parts of their lives. Their realization of what they had initiated and their desire to change often led to monumental trajectory shifts, putting them on healthier, more meaningful life courses.

Seeing all the positive changes and outcomes makes me realize that I can make a profound difference in the lives of others. I am deeply grateful that, for whatever reason, God chose me to play some part in the movement named abortion pill reversal. It has been a distinct privilege to help lead the effort and to be there for women seeking reversals.

I have also been blessed to collaborate with and advise some of the most committed, creative, selfless, excellent clinicians I have ever met. They have gone above and beyond what many expect for physicians and other practitioners, especially in this day of corporate medicine. Always proposing, never imposing, many have been heroic in their efforts to offer APR to women in very challenging circumstances. They have sacrificed time, income, and sometimes professional reputation in order to be there for women seeking a second chance at choice.

I have been equally blessed to work with tireless heroes associated with Culture of Life Family Services, Heartbeat International, and pregnancy help centers all over the country. Many are volunteers who dedicate their lives to helping women and families in crisis pregnancies. Their mentorship, counseling, and simple availability make APR possible and serve as a lifeline for many women who do not have other places to turn.

APR hotline operators and nurses have impressed me to no end. From Vita La Fond to Debbie Bradel, RN, to Liz Delgado, RN, to Christa Brown, RN, they have all been steadfast, selfless, innovative, intrepid, and faithful. They have truly been the warriors in the trenches, doing whatever possible to help women seeking reversal to save their babies. They have made such impressions with their love and dedication that many continue to get text updates with photos of children years after reversals.

The English word *charity* comes from the Latin word *caritas*, which is the translation of the Greek word *agape*. These words all express the love whose aim is doing what is best for others, and APR is truly rooted in this kind of love. It is a movement of medical professionals and people of goodwill seeking to provide whatever assistance is necessary to help women safely and effectively transform the course of death to a pathway that leads to life and love. APR is a metaphor for transformation, forgiveness, redemption, and second chances.

For those who have attempted reversal, whether successful or not, I salute you. I admire your courage and resilience. It can be very difficult to change course in life after making consequential decisions. A person with the insight, fortitude, and faith to accept a second chance at choice is a great person indeed.

For those whose preborn babies died because they were never presented the option of a second chance at choice or chose not to try reversal, I ask you to seek forgiveness and healing. Forgive yourself, for God is merciful and forgiving. Like the prodigal son, we will all be forgiven, as long as we ask.

For men, I have a special message. You are not inconsequential when you have helped conceive a child. You have a role as protector and defender of your partner and your preborn child. Do not shirk your responsibility by defaulting to the current culture's pat line: "I will support whatever choice she makes." Women are more likely to choose life when they know their man will stand by them. Fortitude is a virtue, and modern Western men need to rediscover it.

If you are a man who was involved in an abortion in any way, you likewise need to seek healing and forgiveness. It may be more difficult for men because of the lack of acknowledgment of them in crisis pregnancies and the general marginalization they have experienced in the modern culture.

There are many resources available to help women and men heal. Most local pregnancy help centers have after-abortion counseling. Your local church or congregation may also be a safe place to heal.

Rachel's Vineyard is a nationwide program ready to help. According to its website, "Rachel's Vineyard is a safe place to renew, rebuild and redeem hearts broken by abortion. Weekend retreats offer you a supportive, confidential and non-judgmental environment where women and men can express, release and reconcile painful post-abortive emotions to begin the process of restoration, renewal and healing."[1]

Project Rachel has a list of resources from all over the United States. Additionally, the project has testimonials, prayers, and helpful articles.[2]

Today can be that new day of recovery and renewal. It is there for you to claim, for yourself and for future children, yours and the children of others.

---

[1] "Welcome to Rachel's Vineyard", Rachel's Vineyard, accessed April 10, 2025, https://www.rachelsvineyard.org/.

[2] Project Rachel, accessed April 10, 2025, https://hopeafterabortion.com/.

INDEX

abortifacients, 37, 46, 66
abortion
   activist groups, 182, 206, 219
   as big business, 19, 206. *See also* Big Abortion
   coerced/forced attempted abortions, 65–66
   desensitizing people to, 66–67
   factors influencing decisions about, 17–18
   forgiveness and healing, 240–41
   men and, 240
   Rachel's Vineyard, 158, 241
   resistance and criticism by supporters of, 30, 207, 219–21
   Rh status and, 61–62
   shield laws, 65
   statistics, 37–38, 54–55, 57
abortion industry. *See also* Big Abortion; Medical-Abortion Complex; Planned Parenthood
   ACOG and, 13n, 62, 63, 70, 71, 206
   APR and, 20, 206–10, 224
   growth of, 19
abortion pill. *See also* mifepristone; statistics
   approval in China, 54
   approval in Europe and United States, 54
   Baulieu as developer of, 34–35, 38, 59–60
   as differing from morning-after pill, 37
   generic version of, 51, 221
   marketing of, 39
   politics and, 48–49
   RU-486 as, 23
abortion pill industry
   blurring lines between abortion and contraception by, 66–67
   growth of, 54–58
   Planned Parenthood and, 55–57
   telehealth and mail-order abortions, 60–66
   US government's role, 58–60
abortion pill reversal (APR)
   in Australia, 72–73
   in Canada, 79
   chemical abortion and, 18
   in Colombia, 80–81
   CPR analogy, 20, 215, 225–28
   current state of, 19, 71
   in Europe, 81–82
   evidence supporting, 45–47
   first known reversal, 128–34
   as future standard of care, 20, 71, 235–37
   as ideological threat to Medical-Abortion Complex, 207, 235

abortion pill reversal (APR)
  (*continued*)
  in Israel, 81
  in Lithuania, 79–80
  as metaphor, 20, 240
  in Mexico, 73
  pioneers of, 14, 32
  protocol for, 25, 30n3, 32,
    42, 44–45, 70, 171
  publicity for, 71
  research around, 71
  reversal rate, 42, 44
  in Russia, 73–76
  in Slovenia, 81
  success rate in United
    Kingdom, 188
  in Switzerland, 76–78
  term, 28, 31
  in United Kingdom and
    Ireland, 78–79
  in United States, 68–71
Abortion Pill Rescue Network
  (APRN)
  growth and development
    of, 68
  scope of, 31–32
Abortion Pill Reversal
  Network
  computer map of doctors, 30
  growth and development
    of, 30
  informational website, 28
  launch of, 14, 27
abortion regret, 194, 195,
  209–10
Abortion Rights (UK
  organization), 55
Advancing New Standards
  in Reproductive Health
  (ANSIRH), 209

Allen, Virginia, 223
Alliance Defending Freedom,
  51, 52–53
Alliance for Hippocratic
  Medicine, 52–53
American Academy of Family
  Physicians (AAFP), 13n, 206
American Academy of
  Pediatrics, 50
American Association of
  Pro-Life Obstetricians and
  Gynecologists (AAPLOG),
  29–30, 52–53, 69
American Civil Liberties Union
  (ACLU), 13n, 206, 224
American College of
  Obstetricians and
  Gynecologists (ACOG),
  13n, 62, 63, 70, 71, 158,
  206, 222
American College of
  Pediatricians, 52–53
American Life League (ALL), 64
American Medical Association
  (AMA), 13n, 206
Anzaldo, E. Peter, 44
APR babies
  names of, 20, 197–205
  successful reversals, 26–27
  unsuccessful attempts, 26
Associated Press, 222–23
Australia, 32, 72–73

Baggot, Paddy Jim, 70
Baker, Carrie N., 67
Baptist, Erik, 52–53
Baulieu, Étienne-Émile, 34–35,
  38, 59–60
Belocura, Jonnalyn, 25, 68,
  171–72

Biden administration, 36, 52, 57
Big Abortion. *See also* abortion industry; Medical-Abortion Complex
  APR and, 20, 206–10, 224
  Big Tech and, 219–23
  Creinin study, 210–14
  FDA and, 214–19
  Planned Parenthood and, 56
Big Tech, 219–23
birth defect rate, 42
Bixby Center, 207
Boles, Brent, 69
Bradel, Debbie, 28, 30, 72, 153, 161–66, 239
Brown, Christa, 69, 239
Buffet Foundation, 222
Byrne, Dede, 70

California lawsuits, 53
Calva, Pilar, 73
Canada, 79
Carl, Jerry, 222
Catholic Medical Association (CMA), 29, 71, 177–78, 179, 181
censorship, 219–23
Center for Countering Digital Hate, 219, 221
Centers for Disease Control and Prevention (CDC), 37–38, 219
challenges of APR process
  awareness of APR, 27
  current heroes, 19–20
  for fathers, 19
  finding medical practitioners, 27, 29
  pioneers of APR, 19–20
  for women, 19, 20

Charlotte Lozier Institute, 57
chemical abortion
  alternative terms for, 18
  APR as reversing, 18
  methotrexate reversal, 70
  mifepristone as method for, 33, 35–37
  prevention or reversal debate, 28
  statistics on, 38
  window of opportunity to reverse, 18
China, 54
choice
  common themes when facing, 193–96
  faith and, 195
  gratitude and, 195–96
  regret and, 194, 195, 209
  second chance at, 18, 25, 32, 47, 71, 207, 240
  struggle and turmoil over, 193–94
  support systems and, 194–95
  window of opportunity to reverse, 40
Christian Medical & Dental Associations, 52–53
Citizen Petitions, 51, 52
Clinton administration, 49
Cobb, Leonard, 226
Cohen, Susan A., 59
Colombia, 80–81
Colorado, 224
Commission on Population Growth and the American Future, 59
Complex Family Planning Fellowship, 210

contraception
  abortifacients and, 37, 66
  blurring lines between
    abortion and, 66–67
Corado, Terri, 118–21
COVID-19 pandemic, 36, 52,
  58, 80
CPR analogy, 20, 215,
  225–28
Creinin study, 210–14, 219,
  228
Culture of Life Family Services
  (COLFS), 27, 30, 31, 53,
  68–69, 229, 239

Danco Laboratories, 39, 211,
  221, 222
Davenport, Mary, 26–27, 29,
  43, 69, 209, 212, 230
David and Lucile Packard
  Foundation, 221, 222
De Leon, Rolando, 70
DeBeasi, Paul, 70–71
DeCook, Joseph, 69
Delgado, George
  AAPLOG and, 29–30, 69
  about, 14
  APR and, 238–41
  APRN and, 32
  COLFS and, 53
  first APR case, 167–73
  lawsuit against FDA, 52–53
Delgado, Liz (Elizabeth M.),
  28, 151–60, 239
*Dobbs v. Jackson Women's Health
  Organization*, 57, 220
Duane, Marguerite, 70

ectopic pregnancy, 60, 61, 180,
  188

education
  in CPR, 226
  of health-care professionals,
    29, 81, 230, 234
  of public, 13, 28, 79, 234
emergency medicine
  physicians, 71, 133, 144,
    155, 213, 237
Europe
  abortion kits shipped to, 64
  chemical abortions in, 38, 54
  RU-486 usage in, 23, 39
  study on mifepristone in
    Moldova, 67

false key concept, 35, 132
Family Planning Associates
  (FPA) abortion center, 170
fertilization
  ectopic pregnancy and,
    60–61
  human life and, 9, 60, 67
  in vitro fertilization, 128
Fides et Ratio (1998 encyclical)
  (John Paul II), 230
Foerster, Werner, 44, 77
Fokin, Alexey, 73–76
Food, Drug, and Cosmetic
  Act, 49
Food and Drug Administration
  (FDA)
  2022 lawsuit against, 52–53
  application delays, 214–19,
    233
  approval of generic version
    of mifepristone, 51, 221
  as biased, 13n, 206, 234
  Citizen Petitions against,
    51, 52
  on mifepristone, 46–47

INDEX 247

mifepristone approval,
    48–50, 131
mifepristone regulations, 37,
    168
nonenforcement decision, 52
off-label prescribing, 228
REMS, 50–51
Foster, Angel, 65
France, 39, 54, 60
Francis, Christina, 69
Frost-Clark, Regina, 52–53

Garratt, Debbie, 72–73
GenBioPro, 221
geographical issues, 25, 27, 171
Giles, Angelina, 70
Ginsburg, Ruth Bader, 59
God
    guidance of, 131, 157
    trust in, 20, 172–73
Godsey, Jor-El, 69
Gomperts, Rebecca, 67
Google, 219–21, 222
Goyette, Bill, 30
Graham, Ruth, 235–36
Grauerholz, Kathryn R., 135–50
Grossman, Daniel, 207, 208–9,
    224
guidance
    from COLFS, 30
    from General Medical
        Council (UK), 180
    from God, 131, 157
    offering of, 18
    of Russian Ministry of
        Health, 75
Guttmacher Institute
    abortion statistics, 38, 54, 57
    study on physicians
        performing abortions, 55

Hagan, Rebekah, 114–17
Harrison, Donna, 48–49, 58,
    69, 207
Harrison, Matthew, 14, 19, 26,
    68, 69, 128–34, 230
Hartshorn, Peggy, 69
Hawley, Josh, 220
health departments, need for
    unbiased bureaucrats at, 234
Heartbeat International
    APRN facilitators at, 69
    APRN run by, 68–69, 159,
        229
    booths at conferences by, 29
    heroes of, 239
    lawsuits against, 53
    rebranding as Abortion Pill
        Rescue, 31
Hilgers, Thomas, 14n, 24, 25,
    43, 132
Hoechst AG, 39
hotline
    in Mexico and Latin
        America, 73
    nurses, 19, 28, 69, 135–50,
        151–60, 161–66, 239
    operators, 27, 239
    toll-free number for, 28–29
Hovhannisyan, Tatev, 81–82
human life
    dignity of, 9, 14n, 18, 36–37,
        232–33
    fertilization and, 9, 60, 67
    as gift, 173
Hurm, Sarah, 85–93

Ibis Reproductive Health, 207,
    222
IG Farben, 39–40
in vitro fertilization, 128

infertility, 14n, 24, 132, 201
institutional review board
    (IRB), 31, 41, 215, 216, 217
investigational new drug (IND)
    application, 49, 215–16
Ireland, 78–79
Iriarte, Manrique, 70
Israel, 54, 81

Japan, 45–46
Jester, Shaun, 52–53
John Paul II, Pope Saint, 230
Johnson, Tyler, 52–53

Kearney, Dermot, 19, 78,
    174–89
Kent, Terrence, 72
key analogy, 35, 132
Kliman, Harvey, 178–79,
    235–36
Kouwenhoven, William, 226

La Fond, Vita, 27, 153, 239
Las Libres (group), 64–65
LifeHouse pregnancy center,
    170
LifeSavers Ministries, 169–70,
    171, 172
Lile, William, 70
Lithuania, 79–80
Littlefield, Sarah, 30
Lopez, Roger, 28–29

Maass, Friedrich, 226
Mack, Jonathan, 31
mail-order abortions, 36, 52,
    57, 58, 60–66, 140
mail-order procurement of
    mifepristone, 52
Marchi, Antonio, 63–64

Marcotte, Amanda, 209
Mary Doe (fictitious name),
    124–25
Maxwell, Scott, 30
McCallister, Kelly, 69
medical abortion, 18, 31, 36,
    41, 75, 82. *See also* chemical
    abortion
medical articles
    2018 article, 41–44
    in Australia, 73
    case series study (2018), 30, 41
    by Delgado and Davenport,
        26–27, 41
    peer-review (term), 41
    resistance and criticism of, 30
    withdrawal of, 31
medical professionals. *See also*
    Delgado, George; hotline;
    Kearney, Dermot
    APR physician champions,
        69–70
    in APRN, 68
    banned from saving lives, 19,
        174–89
    nurse practitioners, 135–50
    nurses, 151–60, 161–66
    obstetricians, 71, 237
    physician abortionists, 55–56
    primary care practitioners,
        71, 237
    search for, 29
    targeting of obstetrician
        gynecologists and family
        physicians, 29
Medical-Abortion Complex
    on abortion regrets, 209–10
    abortion/contraception
        distinction and, 66–67
    about, 13–14

APR as ideological threat to, 207, 233, 235–36
brutal reality of, 10
Canada's version of, 79
exploitation of women by, 40
Google censorship and, 221
government's role in development of, 58–60
growing distrust of, 236
organizations of, 13n, 206
Planned Parenthood and, 13n, 56, 206
research bias and, 209, 233
medication abortion, 18, 65. *See also* chemical abortion
Medication Abortion Access Project (MAP), 65
methotrexate reversal, 70
Michel, Cynthia, 100–103
Michel, Jyale, 104–13
Mifegymiso, 23
Mifegyne, 23
Mifeprex, 23
mifepristone. *See also* Food and Drug Administration (FDA); misoprostol; RU-486
abortion process using, 35–37
animal research on, 45–47
blocking of progesterone by, 24–25, 33, 34, 35, 115–16, 131–32
effects of, 34
embryo survival rate after, 42, 43, 45
false key concept, 35, 132
generic version of, 51, 221
history of development as chemical abortion method, 38–40
IND application, 49
lack of proper clinical trials, 49–50
mail-order procurement of, 52
marketing of, 39
morning-after pill comparison to, 37
Pharmacology Review of, 46–47
REMS, 50–51, 52
RU-486 as, 23, 33, 60, 158
Spitz study, 50
statistics on abortions from, 38
US approval of, 39, 48–49, 50
on WHO list of medicines, 48
Mimi (fictitious name), 98–99
miscarriages
APR treatment and, 184, 188, 189
low progesterone levels, 24, 132, 154
prevention of threatened, 163, 171, 237
progesterone and, 179
prostaglandins and, 34
Rh sensitization and, 61
threatened miscarriage defined, 24
treatment of impending, 14, 24, 75
misinformation
at abortion centers, 18
about birth defects, 158
on APR, 219
Heartbeat International and RealOptions Obria Medical Clinics charged with providing, 53

misoprostol
  abortion centers misinformation on, 169, 195
  APR studies and, 218
  availability of, 52, 54, 57–58, 64, 77–78, 176
  coerced/forced attempted abortions and, 63, 65–66
  lack of antidote for, 36, 177, 189
  protocol for, 36
  rare survival after, 170
  as second abortion pill, 43, 115, 130, 143, 168–69, 170, 177
  unlicensed usage of, 179–80
  on WHO list of medicines, 48
Monarres, Angela, 73
Morgan, Carolyn, 72
morning-after pill, 37
My Catholic Doctor, 70
Myrick, Brooke, 69

Nadworny, Elissa, 65
NaProTECHNOLOGY, 14, 25, 132, 151–52, 162
National Abortion Rights Action League (NARAL), 206
National Institute of Child Health and Development (NICHD), 60
National Institutes of Health (NIH), 13n, 45, 60, 206, 234
natural family planning, 128, 132, 162
New York lawsuits, 53

nonenforcement decision, 52
Novielli, Carole, 221–22

Obria Clinic (Orange County, CA), 44
obstetrician gynecologists, 29, 55
Office of Population Research, 58
off-label prescribing, 228
Olohan, Mary Margaret, 223
Open Society Foundations, 206, 221
openDemocracy (group), 182, 221

Palmquist, Terri, 19, 23–26, 167–73
Palmquist, Tim, 167–73
Pariseau, Gabriela, 222
Pediatric Research Equity Act, 49
Pichai, Sundar, 220
Pierre, Lloyd, 70
pill abortion, 18, 28. See also chemical abortion
placebo-controlled trials, 50, 211, 212, 213, 215
placenta
  APR research on cells from, 45
  effects of mifepristone on, 34, 132
  progesterone and, 33–34, 133
  progesterone production by, 25
  separation from uterus, 34, 132, 133, 164
Plan C website, 64, 65

Planned Parenthood
  Guttmacher Institute, 38, 54, 55, 57
  insensitive treatment by, 18, 169
  legal action by, 224
  Medical-Abortion Complex and, 13n, 56, 206
  pro-choice (term), 223
  reference to pill abortions, 28, 55
  revenues from abortion, 55–57, 237
Poehailos, Karen, 70
political agendas. *See also* Big Abortion; Food and Drug Administration (FDA); Medical-Abortion Complex
  blurring lines between abortion and contraception, 66–67
  chemical abortion in United States and, 19
  Democratic Party and push to approve mifepristone, 48–49
  FDA bias, 48–50
  lawsuits against APR providers, 53
  lawsuits against FDA, 52–53
  telehealth and mail-order abortions, 60–66
  US government role in Medical-Abortion Complex, 58–60
  WHO placement of mifepristone and misoprostol on essential medicines list, 48
Population Council, 39, 49, 58–60
preborn babies
  in Creinin study, 211–12
  dignity of, 18
  in ectopic pregnancies, 60
  effects of mifepristone on, 34, 40
  essentials needed for, 33–34
  Rh sensitization and, 62
  safety for, 20
  saved by APR, 18, 19, 47, 68
  survival rate after mifepristone, 42, 212
pregnancy
  FDA's classification as illness, 49
  misdating of, 63
  progesterone as maintaining, 33
pregnancy help centers, 71
  after-abortion counseling at, 241
  medical practitioners from, 29
preterm birth rate, 42
pro-choice (term), 222–23
progesterone
  animal research on, 45–46
  bioidentical progesterone, 14–15, 24, 133
  blocking of, 24–25, 33, 34, 132
  effects on uterus, 34
  emergency room administration of, 237
  as inhibiting production of prostaglandins, 34
  injectable, 25, 43–44
  key analogy, 35, 132

progesterone (*continued*)
　low levels of, 14, 24, 42, 132, 154
　negation of effects of mifepristone, 45, 132
　oral protocol, 43, 44–45
　placenta and, 33–34, 133
　for postpartum depression, 24
　preconception importance of, 33
　in pregnancy, 23, 33
　preterm birth rate and, 42
　to prevent miscarriage, 14, 24, 154, 163
　RU-486 and, 23, 33, 46
　safety of, 227–28
　supplemental, 25, 26–27, 35, 45
　to treat infertility, 24
　uterine lining and, 33
pro-life (term), 222–23
Pro-Life Action Ministries, 170
pro-life advocates
　APR and, 19
　COLFS as, 27
　Helpers of God's Precious Infants, 28–29
　physicians, 29
ProLife Doc, 70
prostaglandins, 34

Rachel's Vineyard, 158, 241
randomized trials, 50, 211, 212, 214–15
Raviele, Kathleen, 70
RealOptions Obria Medical Clinics (San Jose, CA), 53
Reardon, David, 209, 210

regional networks, 32
Reproductive and Placental Research Unit (Yale School of Medicine), 179, 235
research
　on animals, 45–47
　mission to increase, 13
　NIH funding of, 206
　oversight of, 32
Rh sensitization, 61–62
Rich, 126–27
Right to Life Michiana, 63
Risk Evaluation and Mitigation Strategy (REMS), 50–51, 52
Rockefeller, John D., 58, 59
Rockefeller Foundation, 58, 221
Roe v. Wade, 57, 58, 59
Rose, Lila, 220
Roussel Uclaf (RU), 38–39, 48, 49, 60
RU-486. *See also* mifepristone
　ACOG on birth defects and, 158
　approval in Europe and United States, 23
　blocking of progesterone by, 23, 33
　development of, 23, 60
　as developmental label, 38–39
　FDA on abortifacient activity of, 46–47
　mifepristone previously known as, 23, 33, 60
　progesterone and, 23, 33, 46
　Roussel Uclaf and, 38–39, 60
　in Russia, 73–74
Ruberu, Monique, 70

Russia
  APR in, 73–76
  Natasha's story, 122–23
  regional networks in, 32
  RU-486 in, 73–74

Saint Paul VI Institute, 24, 132
Sakiz, Edouard, 39
Sammut, Stephen, 46, 233
Sancta Familia Medical Clinic, 70
Sarai, Emily, 94–97
Sawyer, Allan, 69
Searle, Lisa, 69
shield laws, 65
Slovenia, 81
social media gatekeeping, 219–23
Soros, George, 206, 221
Spitz study, 50
statistical analysis
  in Creinin study, 212, 213, 214
  of reversal rate, 42
statistics
  on abortion, 37–38, 54–55, 57
  on abortion in Europe, 38
  on abortion in United Kingdom, 176
  on abortion pill usage, 131
  on abortion rate for Black women, 59
  on abortion regrets, 210
  on Americans favoring legal abortion, 66
  on APR in United Kingdom, 186–89
  Creinin study and, 212–14
  on ectopic pregnancies, 60
  on medications sent by shield law providers, 65
  on off-label prescribing, 228
  on physicians performing abortions, 55–56
  Planned Parenthood abortions, 56–57
  on reversal rate, 42–43, 44
  on Rh negative population, 61, 62
  on unsuccessful reversals, 165, 188
Steno, Blessed Nicolas, 231–33
Steno Institute, 32, 229–34
surgical abortions
  comparisons to, 40
  in Creinin study, 212, 213
  as irreversible, 18, 177
  Planned Parenthood and, 55
  replacement of, 23, 55–56
Survivor (pamphlet) (Braun), 170
Switzerland, 32, 44, 54, 64, 76–78

telehealth abortions, 36, 57–58, 60–66
Tennessee, 224
Teutsch, George, 38
Tholany, Teresa, 69
Thomas More Society, 53
Toffler, William, 70
Turnaway data, 209–10
Turner, Joseph, 72–73

ultrasounds
  to confirm viability of preborn, 237
  ectopic pregnancy and, 61
  lack of, 63
  refusal to view, 18

United Kingdom
  abortion pill approval in, 54
  APR in, 78–79
  APR success rate in, 188–89
  doctor banned from saving
    lives in, 174–89
  regional networks in, 32
United Nations, 207–8
United States Agency for
  International Development
  (USAID), 13n, 60, 206
University of San Diego
  (USD), 31
US Food and Drug
  Administration (FDA).
  See Food and Drug
  Administration (FDA)
uterine contractions
  effects of mifepristone on, 34
  prostaglandins and, 34

uterine lining
  effects of mifepristone on,
    34, 132
  effects of morning-after pill
    on, 37
  progesterone's role in developing and maintaining, 33

Vance, Ashley, 69
Villinski, Gene, 30

White, Danielle, 69
Women on Waves, 67
World Health Organization
  (WHO), 48, 219

Your Safe Abortion (website), 64

Zuckerberg, Mark, 219
Zyklon B, 40